INTERPROFESSIONAL EDUCATION AND TRAINING

Better partnership working

Series editors: Jon Glasby and Helen Dickinson

About the authors

John Carpenter is Professor of Social Work and Applied Social Science at the University of Bristol, UK, where 30 years ago he designed, ran and evaluated one of the first pre-qualifying programmes of interprofessional education in England. He has since completed comprehensive, longitudinal evaluations of the outcomes of post-qualifying interprofessional education in mental health and a national evaluation of the outcomes of interprofessional and inter-agency training for safeguarding children (child protection).

Helen Dickinson is Associate Professor of Public Governance at the School of Social and Political Sciences and Melbourne School of Government, University of Melbourne, Australia. Her expertise is in public services, particularly in relation to topics such as governance, commissioning and priority setting and decision-making, and she has published widely on these topics. Helen is co-editor of the *Journal of Health, Organization and Management* and the *Australian Journal of Public Administration*. Helen has worked with a range of different levels of government, community organisations and private organisations in Australia, the UK, New Zealand and Europe on research and consultancy programmes.

INTERPROFESSIONAL EDUCATION AND TRAINING

John Carpenter and Helen Dickinson

Second Edition

First edition published in Great Britain in 2008

This edition published in Great Britain in 2016 by

Policy Press
University of Bristol
1-9 Old Park Hill
Bristol BS8 1SD
UK
t: +44 (0)117 954 5940
pp-info@bristol.ac.uk
www.policypress.co.uk

North America office:
Policy Press
c/o The University of Chicago Press
1427 East 60th Street
Chicago, IL 60637, USA
t: +1 773 702 7700
f: +1 773 702 9756
sales@press.uchicago.edu
www.press.uchicago.edu

© Policy Press 2016

British Library Cataloguing in Publication Data
A catalogue record for this book is available from the British Library

Library of Congress Cataloging-in-Publication Data
A catalog record for this book has been requested

ISBN 978-1-4473-2980-0 paperback
ISBN 978-1-4473-2982-4 ePub
ISBN 978-1-4473-2983-1 Mobi

Cover design by Policy Press
Printed and bound in Great Britain by Lavenham Press Ltd, Suffolk
Policy Press uses environmentally responsible print partners

Contents

List of tables, figures and boxes

Tables

Figures

Boxes

Acknowledgements

John and Helen would like to acknowledge the leadership given in the field of interprofessional education (IPE) in the UK by Professor Hugh Barr, and they thank him and his colleagues for allowing them to reproduce the IPE chain reaction illustration (Figure 2.1). John and Helen would also like to thank Sarah Hean and Di Bailey for their helpful comments on the first edition of this book.

Any personal opinions (or errors) in the book are those of the authors.

List of abbreviations

Health and social care use a large number of abbreviations and acronyms. While some of those set out below are fairly popular, the majority pertain to the wide range of technical acronyms that pervade the field of IPE.

AIPHE	Accreditation of Interprofessional Health Education
CAIPE	Centre for the Advancement of Interprofessional Education
CIPW	Creating an Interprofessional Workforce
DH	Department of Health
HCPC	Health and Care Profession Council
HEA	Health Education Authority
HEI	higher education institution
IPE	interprofessional education
IPEC	Interdisciplinary Professional Education Collaboration
JAIPE	Japan Association for Interprofessional Education
MPE	multiprofessional education
NHS	National Health Service
LSCB	Local Safeguarding Children Boards
PBL	problem-based learning
RCT	randomised controlled trial
UPE	uniprofessional education
UWE	University of the West of England
WHO	World Health Organization

All web references in the following text were correct at the time of printing.

A note on terminology

In general, we refer to the people who use services (patients or clients) and to their families (including other non-professional carers) as 'service users and carers'.

We use 'pre-qualifying' to denote all programmes that lead to a professional qualification (or registration). 'Post-qualifying' refers to all educational programmes or training courses for qualified professionals. Post-qualifying educational programmes leading to a university degree may also be referred to as 'postgraduate'. Like others in this field, we do not make a clear distinction between education and training – education programmes are longer than training courses and the latter are generally not assessed, but their aims and methods of learning are often very similar.

Preface

Whenever you talk to people using health and social services, they often assume that the different agencies and professions talk to each other regularly, actively share information and work closely together. Indeed, most people don't distinguish between 'health' and 'social care' at all – or between individual professions such as 'nursing', 'social work' or 'occupational therapy'. They simply have 'needs' that they want addressing in a professional and responsive manner – ideally by someone they know and trust. How the system is structured behind the scenes could not matter less.

And yet, people working in health and social care know that it *does* matter. None of us starts with a blank sheet of paper, and we all have to finds ways of working in a system that was not designed with integration in mind. As the books in this series explain, different parts of our health and social care services have evolved over time as largely separate entities, and policy-makers, managers and front-line practitioners trying to offer a joined-up service will typically face a series of practical, legal, financial and cultural barriers. This is often time-consuming and frustrating, and the end result for service users and their families often still does not feel very integrated (no matter how hard the professionals were working to try to produce a joint way forward). As one key commentator suggests, 'you can't integrate a square peg into a round hole' (Leutz, 1999, p 93).

When services aren't joined-up, it can result in poor outcomes for everybody – gaps, duplication and wasted time and resources. People using services frequently express amazement at the number of different people they have to tell their story to. Instinctively, it doesn't feel like a good use of their time or of the skilled professionals who are trying to help them. Often, one part of the system can't do something until they've had input from another part, and this can lead to all kinds of delays, inefficiencies and missed opportunities.

For staff, it can be surprisingly difficult to find enough time and space to gain a better understanding of how other agencies and professions operate, what they do, what priorities they have and what constraints they face. For someone who went into a caring profession to make a difference, there is nothing more dispiriting than knowing that someone needs a joined-up response but not knowing how to achieve it. In many situations, workers feel they are being asked to help people with complex needs, but with one hand constantly tied behind their back.

For the broader system, this state of affairs seems equally counter-productive. If support is delayed or isn't sufficiently joined-up, it can lead to needs going unmet and to people's health rapidly deteriorating. It then becomes even harder and even more expensive to intervene in a crisis – and this leaves less time and money for other people who are becoming unwell and need support (thus creating a vicious cycle). Poor communication, duplication and arguments over who should pay for what all lead to inefficiency, bad feeling and poor outcomes for people using services. In extreme cases, a lack of joint working can also culminate in very serious, tragic situations – such as a child death, a mental health homicide, the abuse of a person with learning difficulties or an older person dying at home alone (see Box 0.1 for but one high profile example). Here, partnership working is quite literally a matter of life and death, and failure to collaborate can have the most serious consequences for all involved.

Box 0.1: Partnership working as a matter of life or death

Following the tragic death of Peter Connelly (initially known as 'Baby P' in the press), Lord Laming (2009) was asked to produce a national review of progress since his initial investigation into the equally horrific death of Victoria Climbié in the same borough of Haringey (Laming, 2003). As the 2009 review observed (Laming, 2009, para 4.3):

> It is evident that the challenges of working across organisational boundaries continue to pose barriers in practice, and that cooperative efforts are often the first to suffer when services and individuals are under pressure. Examples of poor practice highlighted to this report include child protection conferences where not all the services involved in a child's life are present or able to give a view; or where one professional disagrees with a decision and their view is not explored in more detail; and repeated examples of professionals not receiving feedback on referrals. As a result of each of these failures, children or young people at risk of neglect or abuse will be exposed to greater danger. The referring professional may also be left with ongoing anxiety and concern about the child or young person. This needs to be addressed if all local services are to be effective in keeping children and young people safe.

For health and social care practitioners, if you are to make a positive and practical difference to service users and patients, most of the issues you face will involve working with other professions and other organisations. For public service managers, partnership working is likely to occupy an increasing amount of your time and budget, and arguably requires different skills and approaches to those prioritised in traditional single agency training and development courses. For social policy students and policy-makers, many of the issues you study and/ or try to resolve inevitably involve multiple professions and multiple organisations. Put simply, people do not live their lives according to the categories we create in our welfare services – real-life problems are nearly always messier, more complex, harder to define and more difficult to resolve than this.

Policy context

In response, national and local policy increasingly calls for enhanced and more effective partnership working as a potential solution (see, for example, DH, 2013). While such calls for more joint working can be inconsistent, grudgingly made and/or overly aspirational, the fact remains that collaboration between different professions and different organisations is increasingly seen as the norm (rather than as an exception to the rule). This is exemplified in a previous Welsh policy paper, *The sustainable social services for Wales: A framework for action* (Welsh Assembly Government, 2011, p 11) that argued, 'We want to change the question from "how might we cooperate across boundaries?" to justifying why we are not.' With most new funding and most new policy initiatives, there is usually a requirement that local agencies work together to bid for new resources or to deliver the required service, and various Acts of Parliament place statutory duties of partnership on a range of public bodies. As an example of the growing importance of partnership working, in 1999 the word 'partnership' was recorded 6,197 times in official parliamentary records, compared to just 38 times in 1989 (Jupp, 2000, p 7). When we repeated this exercise for the first edition of this book, we found 17,912 parliamentary references to 'partnership' in 2006 alone (although this fell to 11,319 when removing references to legislation on civil partnerships that was being debated at the time). Since then, there have been two general elections/ new governments and a series of major spending cuts and pressures – arguably making joint working harder to achieve in practice, but even more important.

In 1998, the Department of Health issued a consultation document on future relationships between health and social care. Entitled *Partnership in action*, the document proposed various ways of promoting more effective partnerships, basing these on a scathing but extremely accurate critique of single agency ways of working:

> All too often when people have complex needs spanning both health and social care good quality services are sacrificed for sterile arguments about boundaries. When this happens people, often the most vulnerable in our society ... and those who care for them find themselves in the no man's land between health and social services. This is not what people want or need. It places the needs of the organisation above the needs of the people they are there to serve. It is poor organisation, poor practice, poor use of taxpayers' money – it is unacceptable. (DH, 1998, p 30)

Whatever you might think about subsequent policy and practice, the fact that a government document sets out such a strongly worded statement of its beliefs and guiding principles is important. How to move from the rhetoric to reality is always the key challenge – but such quotes illustrate that partnership working is no longer an option (if it ever was), but core business. Under the coalition government (2010-15), this previous language shifted once again – and most recent policy refers to the importance of 'integrated care' (rather than 'partnerships' or 'collaboration'). As the coalition's NHS Future Forum (2012, p 3) argued:

> Integration is a vitally important aspect of the experience of health and social care for millions of people. It has perhaps the greatest relevance for the most vulnerable and those with the most complex and long-term needs. We have services to be proud of, and patients in England already receive some of the most joined-up services in the world. However, too many people fall through gaps between services as they traverse journeys of care which are often too difficult for them to navigate themselves. This lack of integration results daily in delays and duplication, wasted opportunities and

patient harm. It is time to "mind the gaps" and improve the experience and outcomes of care for people using our services.

While it is not always fully clear what a commitment to more integrated care might mean in practice (see below for further discussion), recent policy seems to be trying to achieve a number of different things, including:

- greater *vertical integration* between acute, community and primary care
- greater *horizontal integration* between community health and social care
- more effective joint working between *public health* and local government
- more effective partnerships between the *public, private and voluntary sectors*
- more *person-centred care*, with services that feel integrated to the patient.

In response to all this, the time feels right for a second edition of this book and of our 'Better partnership working' Series more generally. While our overall approach remains the same (see below for a summary of our aims and ethos), key changes to this edition include:

- updated references to current policy and practice
- the addition of more recent studies and broader literature
- a greater focus on 'integrated care' under the coalition government (2010-15) and the Conservative government of 2015-
- new reflective exercises and updated further reading/resources
- updated 'hot topics' (with a particular focus in some of the books in the series on the importance of working together during a time of austerity).

Aims and ethos

Against this background, this book (and the overall series of which it is part) provides an introduction to partnership working via a series of accessible 'how to' resources (see Box 0.2). Designed to be short and easy to use, they are nevertheless evidence-based and theoretically robust. A key aim is to provide *rigour and relevance* via books that:

- offer practical support to those working with other agencies and professions and to provide some helpful frameworks with which to make sense of the complexity that partnership working entails;
- summarise current policy and research in a detailed but accessible manner;
- provide practical but also evidence-based recommendations for policy and practice.

Box 0.2: The series at a glance

- *Partnership working in health and social care* (Jon Glasby and Helen Dickinson, 2nd edn)
- *Managing and leading in inter-agency settings* (Helen Dickinson and Gemma Carey, 2nd edn)
- *Interprofessional education and training* (John Carpenter and Helen Dickinson, 2nd edn)
- *Working in teams* (Kim Jelphs, Helen Dickinson and Robin Miller, 2nd edn)
- *Evaluating outcomes in health and social care* (Helen Dickinson and Janine O'Flynn, 2nd edn)

While each book is cross-referenced with others in the series, each is a standalone text with all you need to know as a student, practitioner, manager or policy-maker to make sense of the difficulties inherent in partnership working. In particular, the series aims to provide some practical examples to illustrate the more theoretical knowledge of social policy students, and some theoretical material to help make sense of the practical experiences and frustrations of front-line workers and managers.

Although there is a substantial literature on partnership working (see, for example, Hudson, 2000; Payne, 2000; Rummery and Glendinning, 2000; Balloch and Taylor, 2001; 6 et al, 2002; Glendinning et al, 2002; Sullivan and Skelcher, 2002; Barrett et al, 2005; Glasby and Dickinson, 2014a, for just some of many potential examples), most current books are either broad edited collections, very theoretical books that are inaccessible for students and practitioners, or texts focusing on partnership working for specific user groups. Where more practical, accessible and general texts exist, these typically lack any real depth or evidence base – in many ways, they are little more than partnership 'cookbooks' that give apparently simple instructions that are meant to lead to the perfect and desired outcome. In practice, anyone who has studied or worked in health and social care knows that partnership working can be both frustrating and messy – even if you follow the so-called 'rules', the end result is often hard to predict, ambiguous and likely to provoke different reactions from different agencies and professions. In contrast, this book series seeks to offer a more 'warts and all' approach to the topic, acknowledging the realities that practitioners, managers and policy-makers face in the real world.

Wherever possible, the series focuses on key concepts, themes and frameworks rather than on the specifics of current policy and organisational structures (which inevitably change frequently). As a result, the series will hopefully be of use to readers in all four countries of the UK as well as other national settings. That said, where structures and key policies have to be mentioned, they will typically be those in place in England.

While the focus of the series is on public sector health and social care, it is important to note from the outset that current policy and practice also emphasises a range of additional partnerships and relationships, including:

- broader partnerships (for example, with services such as transport and leisure in adult services and with education and youth justice in children's services);
- collaboration not just between services, but also between professionals and people who use services;
- relationships between the public, private and voluntary sectors.

As a result, many of the frameworks and concepts in each book may focus initially on public sector health and social care, but will also be relevant to a broader range of practitioners, students, services and service users.

Ultimately, the current emphasis on partnership working and on integration means that everything about public services – their organisation and culture, professional education and training, inspection and quality assurance – will have to change. Against this background, we hope that this series of books is a contribution, however small, to these changes.

Jon Glasby and Helen Dickinson
University of Birmingham and University of Melbourne
December 2015

1

What is interprofessional education and why does it matter?

Collaborative working has assumed an important role within UK public services over the past 30 years, with successive national governments viewing greater inter-agency working as crucial to driving good government. But an awareness of the need for professions in medicine, health and social care to work together more effectively has been around for much longer, and not only in the UK (WHO, 1998). The idea that professionals should 'learn together to work together' – what has come to be called 'interprofessional education' (IPE) – is not a new idea by any means (for further discussion on this, see Szasz, 1969; Baldwin, 1996). Nevertheless, interest in this concept has grown dramatically over the last 15 years or so. As Barr et al (2011, p 5) argue,

> The turn of the Century was a watershed in the short history of ... IPE ... in the UK ... when the Labour government promoted "common learning" to be built in to the mainstream of pre-registration professional education for all the health and social care professions to help implement its modernisation strategy.... The proposition was as seductive as it was simple: learning together would deliver not only a more collaborative but also a more flexible and more mobile workforce responsive to the exigencies of practice and the expectations of management.

As this quote illustrates, IPE has been perceived as one potential solution to a number of the practical difficulties associated with collaborative working. Health and social care collaborations bring together a range of different professions ostensibly to work together around the needs of service users. However, professions often have different values and perspectives underpinning the delivery of care and informing the ways in which they view other professions. IPE is seen as a way to overcome ignorance and prejudice between health and social care professionals. By learning together, it is argued, professions will better understand each other and value what others bring to the practice of collaboration. It is often proposed that ultimately, through working together more effectively, this will improve the quality of care and outcomes for service users.

The converse of this is also suggested: not learning together is thought to have a negative impact on services and service users. High-profile inquiries have consistently cited poor inter-agency and interprofessional working as a contributing factor towards failure on behalf of particular service users, and recommendations for IPE have been made as a result. IPE is regarded as crucial within particular areas such as safeguarding children, community mental health services, older people's services, services for disabled children and other such contexts where it is suggested that vulnerable people – often with quite high levels of need – will only receive quality of care if services are delivered by professionals who understand each other's roles and responsibilities, so that care can be coordinated. In many cases, multiprofessional teams (also called multidisciplinary teams) provide such care. However, IPE is not restricted just to these areas of service delivery. There is also a growing interest in using IPE to improve multidisciplinary teamworking within settings such as hospitals, community-based teams and, to some degree, primary care.

This second edition of the book has been revised to reflect the advances that have been made in the theory and practice of IPE since the first edition. Updates have been made to the policy context and new research has been incorporated, with an emphasis on new systematic reviews of the sustainability of IPE and the outcomes of IPE. In particular we reflect on the growth of IPE internationally, and have included summaries of developments in Norway, Canada, the US,

Japan and Australia, and examples of programmes outside the UK. The contribution of social psychological theory to programme planning has been extended in light of recent work.

Despite – or perhaps because of – the current interest in IPE, there are a number of prefixes (multi/inter/uni/trans), adjectives (professional/ disciplinary) and nouns (education/training/learning/studies) that are married together in any number of ways to refer to a range of phenomena that fit broadly within this area. Each of these terms has a different meaning, but there is a tendency to use them inconsistently. McCallin (2001, p 421) suggests that this irregularity of usage is causing difficulties in terms of definition: 'overall ... descriptions in the professional literature are so diverse that meaning is murky'. To aid clarification, this chapter starts with an overview of a range of key terms that might be encountered when reading about and discussing IPE. We then go on to provide a brief exploration of the historical and policy context, examining where interest in IPE has developed from, and how it has an impact on health and social care practitioners. The chapter concludes by considering the aims of IPE, the forms it may take and some of the key theories that might underpin it. The following chapters then build on this overview in more detail. The text draws on evidence of good and bad practice throughout, and presents a number of case studies and examples of the types of materials that have been used in IPE. The intention is that the text will offer practical – yet rigorous and relevant – evidence and advice on how to initiate, run and evaluate IPE.

Key terms

In the introductory text in this series by Jon Glasby and Helen Dickinson (2014b) a range of terms are examined that relate to the 'partnership' phenomenon and associated definitions. The field of IPE suffers a similar fate to that of 'partnership' in that, as noted above, and reiterated by a range of commentators, 'interprofessional education is bedevilled by terminological inexactitude' (Barr et al, 2005, p xvii). Many different terms are used within the broad field of IPE, often interchangeably and inaccurately. But these terms are underpinned by different values and associated expectations and rationales. Some of those more frequently used are defined in Box 1.1 below, but this is by no means an exhaustive list. The key definition of interprofessional education is that used by Zwarenstein et al (2000) in the first – and succeeding – Cochrane reviews of research on this subject, and this is included in Box 1.1.

Box 1.1: Helpful definitions

- *Uniprofessional education (UPE):* occasions when professionals or students from one profession learn together.
- *Multiprofessional education (MPE) (or learning):* occasions when two or more professions learn side by side in parallel.
- *Interprofessional education (IPE):* occurs when members of more than one health and/or social care profession learn interactively together, for the explicit purpose of improving interprofessional collaboration and/or the health and wellbeing of patients or clients. Interactive learning requires active learner participation and active exchange between learners from the different professions (Zwarenstein et al, 2000).
- *Transprofessional education:* occasions in real practice where professional boundaries have been crossed or merged.
- *Shared learning:* similar to multiprofessional learning, where students or professionals learn alongside each other, but do not necessarily interact.
- *Common learning:* a term previously used by the Department of Health (DH) in England, which suggests that health and social care students should, in part, follow a common curriculum.

An important point to elaborate here is the distinction between IPE and MPE – IPE promotes collaborative practice between professions, while MPE is simply learning together for whatever reason, including, for example, economies of scale in which health professionals share lectures on topics of mutual interest. Although a seemingly semantic differentiation, the intent behind the purposes of MPE and IPE programmes are different, which in turn has important implications for determining content, teaching methods and evaluation.

Looking internationally, the World Health Organization (WHO, 2010, p 5) has been influential in promoting IPE, and defines IPE as occurring 'when two or more professions learn about, from and with each other to enable effective collaboration and improve health outcomes.' This definition is indistinguishable from that of IPE in Box 1.1, although it is important to note that the WHO's definition does not just involve professions learning alongside each other, but also collaborating. In the UK, the Centre for the Advancement of Interprofessional Education (CAIPE) (1996) suggests that IPE is a subset of MPE, set apart by its purpose and methods. In other words, MPE is an overarching approach to education, of which IPE is a more specialised branch for particular purposes.

In practice, this means that we need to be clear about how we are using terms such as MPE or IPE, and that others also understand this. We cannot presume that all other stakeholders will interpret these concepts in the way we intend, and we should be explicit at the outset of any discussions.

Given the terminological difficulties and a recent expansion of IPE activities, a number of commentators have expressed a concern that IPE is weak in terms of setting out its aims and also the learning theories that underpin programmes. In order to be clearer about what IPE should entail, Barr (2002, p 23) produced a definition of IPE aims and methods that has now become quite widely used. Barr identifies the components of IPE as:

> The application of principles of adult learning to interactive, group-based learning, which relates collaborative learning to collaborative practice within a coherent rationale which is informed by understanding of interpersonal, group, organisational and inter-organisational relations and processes of professionalisation. (Barr, 2002, p 23)

In other words, IPE should be more specific than just professions undertaking collaborative learning, but should be underpinned by a clear sense of why such a programme is being pursued and the theories that underpin this learning. Moreover, this definition also stresses that the ultimate intention of IPE is to improve collaborative practice, rather than be an end in itself (much as this series has tried to stress that collaborative working should be about specific improvement aims and objectives rather than simply an aim in itself).

History and policy background

As Barr (2002) notes, the UK IPE movement began in the 1960s as a series of discrete and predominantly local initiatives that often had differing motivations behind their establishment. These were either specific to geographic areas or challenges, or else allied with particular professions, which generally meant that IPE was viewed as important for different reasons. These early initiatives were often reactive, isolated and relatively short-lived. However, over time, education providers became more proactive and less remedial in their approaches, and we started to see postgraduate-level programmes designed more or less explicitly to promote interprofessional collaboration among qualified practitioners.

The NHS Plan (DH, 2000a) really ignited national interest in the importance of different professional groups working together to 'modernise' services. This document refers to one of the underlying problems of the National Health Service (NHS) being 'old-fashioned demarcations between staff and barriers between services', and calls for a modernised seamless service designed 'around the needs of the patient' (DH, 2000a, p 10). It refers not only to barriers between NHS services, but also to barriers between the NHS and local government (in particular, social care).

As the demands of society have changed with an ageing population and an increased emphasis on the long-term management of chronic illness, multiprofessional teamwork is seen as a way of enabling service users to receive a professionally coordinated and comprehensive plan of care from a range of providers (Barr et al, 2011). Education and training are an important way in which students and professionals can be better equipped to take on this role. *The NHS Plan* stated that a new 'core curriculum' would be introduced into education programmes for NHS staff, and a common foundation programme would allow students and staff to switch careers and training paths more easily (DH, 2000a, p 86). This document also makes reference to the potential for some professions (for example, nurses) to widen their remit and to take on a much broader role spanning professions. Education and training is therefore not only seen as a way to modernise services and provide them around the needs of service users, but also to change the nature of the workforce. However, the only elements of the core curriculum referred to are communication skills and learning about NHS principles and organisation, and *The NHS Plan* was not explicit about the precise form that this education and training should take.

The principles of *The NHS Plan* were taken forward in a further series of documents that reaffirmed the government's interest in IPE (DH, 2001a, 2002a). These documents suggested that all health professionals should expect to have common learning with other professionals at each stage of their learning and training from pre-qualification to continuing professional development. These programmes should be flexible and provide modules with common and core skills. The aim was that common learning would be a reality for all pre-qualifying students by 2004. These reforms were laid out in papers that addressed specific health and social care disciplines (see, for example, DH, 1999, 2000b, 2002b). Furthermore, workforce planning documents (see, for example, DH, 2001b, 2002c) have generally enforced this approach, calling for more flexible working and changes in roles and functions. They suggest a need for more responsive services and planning across clinical, local authority and voluntary sector services, but recognise that achieving these aims will require fundamental changes to workforce and practice development, and a number highlight the importance of IPE in delivering these improvements.

As Barr et al (2011) outline in their review of IPE in the UK, there have been frequent policy shifts over successive governments, but in practice these have redrawn the occupational map 'less than might have been expected, reflecting the power of professional institutions to preserve the status quo and awareness of the need to restrict title, preserve professional demarcations and specify responsibilities to improve patient safety' (2011, p 10). Indeed, a number of high-profile enquiries into deaths and poor care (see, for example, DH, 2001c; Laming, 2003, 2009) have noted the contribution that failures of inter-agency working have made to these events, but frequent reorganisations have often destabilised working relationships, throwing professionals into a defensive mode, meaning that it is less likely that they will collaborate just as they need to. This has made the need for IPE even starker as a way to help 'preserve and sometimes repair relationships' (Barr et al, 2011, p 10). A report into patient safety from the House of Commons Health Committee (2009, para 290), for example, argued that there were 'convincing arguments for interdisciplinary training to foster good teamwork skills across professional boundaries: those who work together should train together.'

In England, Local Safeguarding Children Boards (LSCBs) have a legal responsibility for ensuring that all health, local authorities, the police and voluntary organisations cooperate to safeguard and promote the welfare of children in their area; this includes the provision of inter-agency training, specifically to promote and develop shared understanding of roles and responsibilities, and effective working relationships. Extensive training programmes have been organised, typically of courses lasting one to two days. Following the guidance, courses are on three levels: from introductory courses on definitions, policies and procedures for those in contact with children, to specialist courses on topics such as interprofessional practice to safeguard disabled children and children living in families with domestic violence. Participants include community nurses, social workers, doctors, specialist teachers, and the police, among others (HM Government, 2010).

A review of IPE in the UK from 1997-2013 (see Barr et al, 2014) surmises that many of the forces in driving IPE have been external in the form of government policies, funding and findings from inquiries into failures of care. As a consequence of this, during the early years of the 2000s, substantial funding was made available to make 'major steps forward, especially in scaling up IPE, but infrastructures set up were vulnerable to disbandment when the funding ceased' (Barr et al, 2014, p 10).

Teaching and learning about interprofessional practice have been made specific curricula requirements in subject benchmark statements from the Quality Assurance Agency (QAA). These statements set out expectations about standards and content of degrees in a range of subject areas, including degrees in nursing, allied health and social work.

The UK has not been alone in developing IPE approaches, and Barr (2015) sets out an overview of IPE initiatives that have been developed in a variety of countries. We summarise below some of the most interesting examples from around the world in Box 1.2. These illustrate many of the themes about developing and sustaining IPE presented in the next chapter.

Box 1.2: International development of IPE

Norway

As in the UK, health and social care services were criticised by government through the 1980s and 1990s for a lack of collaboration. A greater focus on collaborative skills and teamwork were identified as being important in terms of professional education. Influenced by international trends, a common learning curriculum was developed with four elements: science and research methods, ethics, communication and societal structures (Barr, 2015). This common core would involve multi- or interdisciplinary learning to enhance collaborative practice, although this was only partially implemented. Most universities did not see the value of interprofessional learning, while others struggled logistically in terms of combining curricula or because of the number of small learning institutions that only educated one professional group and therefore lacked opportunities for interprofessional learning. As we outline later in Chapter 3, a lack of university leadership around IPE has often been a challenge for embedding this in English universities.

In 2012 the Norwegian government published a white paper on education for health and social care, outlining the importance of IPE for professionals to gain collaborative competences. Although some universities had developed common interprofessional learning units within health and social care programmes, this was rather piecemeal. The white paper recommended that there should be IPE during placements, and a national planning group was established to develop a proposal on the common core.

Canada

The first IPE initiative in Canada was developed by the University of British Columbia in the 1960s, driven by the idea that health and social care professions needed to be educated together. Activities included seminars, field trips, clinical experiences and interviews (Szasz, 1969), and the effects seemed largely promising. However, they ran into serious challenges in the early 1970s as a result of changes to the regulation of professional courses and, echoing the Norwegian experience, a lack of university support for the ideas.

It was another 30 years before the Romanow Commission (2002) called for new models of training to help implement new care models. The federal government launched the Interprofessional Education for Collaborative Patient-Centred Practice that sought to promote IPE and its benefits, increase the number of health professionals trained through IPE and share best practice in educating for collaborative practice. Substantial financial resources were made available over five years for developments in IPE and collaborative practice (Herbert, 2005). Research was developed to underpin this process (D'Amour and Oandasan, 2005), and evaluation was seen as essential to the programmes. As we will further discuss in Chapter 3, dedicated resources distributed according to sound evidence-based approaches and underpinned by evaluative practice are important drivers in sustaining IPE.

Between 2006 and 2012 the federal government funded the Canadian Interprofessional Health Collaborative (CIHC) that facilitated exchange and support around IPE developments in Canada and also with the US. This has continued as a third sector organisation, hosted by the University of British Columbia. The International Association for Interprofessional Education and Collaborative Practice was formed, and was central to the work of the WHO (2010). Significant developments followed with the formulation of national interprofessional core competencies (CIHC and CPIS, 2010) and the Accreditation of Interprofessional Health Education (AIPHE) initiative. Core principles concerning language, context, evidence and criteria were embedded in the AIPHE to be implemented by local organisations. This seeks to improve consistency between member organisations and ensure a common approach that will still have a degree of local flexibility. Again, we talk about the importance of this in developing sustainable IPE in the following chapter.

USA

Like Canada, IPE programmes started early in the US (Baldwin, 1996). During the 1970s, six medical schools – Nevada, Michigan State, North Carolina, Washington, Utah and California at San Francisco – devised a common model for team training (Barr, 2015). While most of these IPE programmes had university and work-based initiatives, they varied in their focus and approach. Kuehn (1998) argues that IPE rose in importance in the 1990s as a response to the rising costs of health services and the education of professionals. The Pew Health Professions' Commission outlined the series of changes that would be needed in relation to education processes in order to match the changes happening in the US health system. An important part of these recommendations was a requirement for all health professionals to have an interdisciplinary competence.

The impetus for IPE was further secured following the Institute of Medicine's report into avoidable deaths within health services (Kohn et al, 1999). Interdisciplinary teams were identified as one of five core learning areas for all health professions students (IOM, 2003). The Institute for Healthcare Improvement developed the Interdisciplinary Professional Education Collaborative (IPEC), which agreed core competences for interprofessional collaborative practice to guide the development of curriculums in all health professional schools (Interprofessional Education Collaborative Expert Panel, 2011). Again, this illustrates the importance of a collective approach to guidance for the development of curricular that establishes a core, but which is flexible to local needs.

As this overview of the US experience has suggested so far, unlike some other countries where the IPE agenda has been firmly driven by government, philanthropic foundations have played an important role in promoting IPE. (In the 'Further reading' section at the end of the chapter we provide links to some of these initiatives.) An important activity that many of these organisations have been involved in has been the need to develop high-quality research relating to collaboration, teamwork and IPE. Although intuitively it seems that IPE should improve collaborative practice and outcomes, reviews of the US literature have been unable to demonstrate this link empirically (Brandt et al, 2014). Nevertheless, the frequency of adverse events from medical errors and calls for improvement continue to demand more IPE activity.

Japan

As in the US, interest in Japan has been attributed to concerns regarding quality of healthcare and inadequate quality assurance (Watanabe and Koizumi, 2010). A number of critical incidents brought these issues to the attention of the public, fuelled by reports of child abuse cases and the suicide of a celebrity. The Japanese government funded IPE initiatives that were incorporated into professional education. Exchanges with UK and Canadian universities were developed to learn from international experience, which, we argue in the next chapter, is crucial in developing sustainable programmes of IPE. Chiba University was designated by the government as the lead interprofessional research institution and Gunma University as a WHO interprofessional centre (Makino et al, 2012). The Japan Association for Interprofessional Education (JAIPE) was also launched in 2008 to provide a forum for exchange between university staff and professionals focusing on key areas of health and social care practice (Takahashi and Kinoshita, 2015).

As of 2008 more than half the medical schools were implementing IPE, but on the whole, implementation was uneven between different universities and professions. The Consortium for Interprofessional Education won central government funding to develop a number of IPE modules based on interprofessional teamworking to problem solve, and the CAIPE principles (Barr and Low, 2012) were used as the starting point for this.

Australia

One of Australia's first IPE programmes was developed in Sydney in the 1970s, and plans were made at the time for IPE at 10 different medical schools. However, only one of these emerged, at the University of Adelaide, where federal funding enabled a joint programme for 600 undergraduate students across community health practice. As we will argue in the following chapter, working collaboratively with community partners has often proved to be a helpful way in which to develop sustainable IPE. In this case, funding was withdrawn in the late 1980s, but the programme did continue, and indeed expanded to other institutions and professions.

Developments took place in a number of other Australian universities underpinned by some sort of common curriculum, although there was often a lack of flexibility to develop these courses (Graham and Wealthall, 1999, in Barr et al, 2015). A number of reviews confirmed that the development of IPE had been localised, opportunistic, adaptive and creative on the margins of existing curricula. Resources invested had been minimal and developments, as a consequence, frequently unsustainable. Nevertheless, there was strong support in higher education, health and government.

In a report to the government office of higher education, a consortium of universities examined what was necessary for IPE to progress as a coherent and well-coordinated national project (Steketee, 2014). A wide range of conceptual and practical resources was developed for shaping, delivering, assessing and evaluating IPE. Of particular importance was a 'four dimensional curriculum development framework'. IPE has become an explicit focus for government, with funding made available for the development of a 'national IPE work plan' (Dunston et al, 2015). This was intended to set out a national approach incorporating curriculum and standards development, knowledge management, capacity and support and national leadership. The work plan proposes a National Leadership

Council that would promote the principles, values, development and visibility of IPE at the most senior level in higher education, health service provision, the professions, educational standards, health professions' regulation, safety and quality, and continuing professional development.

The key point from the comparison of IPE initiatives set out above and based on Barr (2015) is that one size does not fit all and difference should be celebrated rather than feared. Yet the conclusion reached is that 'much remains to be done to develop institutions and infrastructure for the emerging global interprofessional movement, but the foundations are being laid' (Barr, 2015, p 38). Reflecting back on the recent history since the publication of the first edition of this book, it seems that there has been significant and ongoing activity over this period, although of a different quantum to the momentum through the first decade of this century. As this field evolves the question remains whether this work has had a substantial impact in practice, and for this we need to revisit what it is precisely that IPE is seeking to deliver.

Aims of IPE

Examining the policy background and trajectory of IPE is more than simply an instructive history lesson. What this brief overview of policy and government initiatives suggests is that IPE has moved from being a relatively marginal part of the health and social care educational system to playing quite a central role within post-qualifying education and training. Yet, despite moving into more central territory, health and social care IPE is still underpinned by a range of different motivations. Finch (2000, p 1138), writing as a university vice chancellor, suggested that students need to be prepared for interprofessional working in a number of senses:

- to *know about* the roles of other professional groups;
- to be able to *work with* the roles of other professionals, in the context of a team where each member has a clearly defined role;

- to be able to *substitute for* roles traditionally played by other professionals, when circumstances suggest that this would be more effective;
- to provide *flexibility* in career routes (moving across).

The policy history set out in the previous section suggested roles for IPE in supporting some – if not all – of these goals. We are interested here in the role of IPE in preparing students of different professions for working together as practitioners, and subsequently in supporting and developing collaborative working between professionals in health and social care organisations. Also, as the teamworking text in this series suggests (see Jelphs et al, 2016), IPE can make an important contribution to developing more effective multiprofessional teamwork in inter-agency settings.

Before deciding on the content and structure of any IPE programme, it is important that we are clear exactly what it is that we want from it. Every programme should start by asking the question, what are we really trying to achieve by delivering a programme of IPE to a particular group? Aims should be outlined in a clear and concise manner, obviously demonstrating why IPE is necessary for this programme of education or training. As we will demonstrate throughout, IPE is not easy to do (when it is done well), and so if you don't need to do it (or aren't going to do it properly), then you might want to consider a different approach. Whatever approach is selected should be determined by the purpose. This is seemingly an obvious point, but as reflected above, this has not always been apparent in IPE initiatives. Barr (2002, p 6) observes:

> Interprofessional education has been invoked ever more frequently during the past thirty years to encourage collaboration in health and social care to help improve services, effect change and, latterly, implement workforce strategies. Expectations have been raised and objectives added with each succeeding wave of development, introduced for other reasons unsupported by adequate argument and evidence caught up in wider moves towards shared learning. Definition has

been lacking, semantics bewildering, evaluations few and
the evidence base elusive. Small wonder teachers are uneasy.

IPE has become more and more popular, and has been seen as a
potential solution to help overcome a range of difficulties. In one
sense this has been positive as IPE has gained recognition within a
wide range of different fields. However, this also means that IPE runs
the risk of being seen as all things to all people (there are interesting
parallels here with the notion of collaboration itself – more of which
later). IPE has also been criticised for lacking 'conceptual clarity'
and consequently of being merely a trend in health and social care
education (Campbell and Johnson, 1999). Without a sense of precision
over what IPE is aiming to achieve, and without being underpinned
by explicit and appropriate content and theory, the concept of IPE
risks losing legitimacy. This is not to say that IPE might not be able to
support improvement in all the areas that Finch outlines (2000), but it
is unlikely that any one programme would achieve such a broad range
of objectives simultaneously (see Chapter 3 for a further discussion
of IPE and outcomes).

Clearly, the achievement of some objectives requires organisational
change as well as education. For example, even if nursing and medical
students learned new ways of collaborating in which nurses were able to
substitute for doctors' roles in some respects, this would be insufficient
if senior doctors, or patients for that matter, rejected this on principle.
Therefore, when embarking on the design of an IPE programme it
is important to consider what it is precisely that you are aiming to
achieve with that particular initiative, that this is realistic in the sense
that IPE is actually capable of making these changes, and which other
stakeholder groups might need to be involved in this process.

Forms of IPE

As demonstrated above, IPE programmes can have rather different aims,
and so it follows that there are a range of different forms that it might
take. Expanding on this notion, Barr (1996) identifies a number of

different dimensions of IPE (see Box 1.3). Specific choices relating to these dimensions will need to be made with consideration of the aims of the IPE programme clearly in mind. For example, if the aim of IPE is to help a group of practitioners from different professions initiate a quality improvement programme to produce a particular change, it is unlikely that it will be effective if designed with an individual, college-based, didactic format. Similarly, if the programme is in the early days of a pre-qualifying course, it is unlikely to be implicit, all of a programme, or delivered in a purely work-based setting. Indeed, a fundamental distinction is between pre-qualifying IPE, which has the aim of preparing students to work together and which is organised by higher education institutions (HEIs), and post-qualifying IPE, which aims to improve partnership practice and which is generally shorter and employment-based.

Box 1.3: Barr's (1996) dimensions of IPE

- *Implicit or explicit:* IPE might go unrecognised in everyday work or may occur through serendipitous multiprofessional learning (that is, learning as an inadvertent consequence of bringing professionals together). This learning is implicit and may be consolidated and verified when it is made explicit. Explicit IPE is often through courses, workshops and conferences.
- *Discrete or integrated:* IPE might be freestanding modules designed to improve quality of care through better collaboration or integrated into other MPE or UPE as a specific area of learning.
- *All or part of a programme:* IPE might be the entirety of a programme or just an aspect of it. It is unlikely to ever be the whole of a pre-qualification course, although it could be all of a post-qualification programme.
- *General or particular:* IPE may concentrate on a particular user group, method or setting, or be more broadly based.
- *Positive or negative:* IPE might have a positive impact on relationships and collaborative work, but there is also the potential for a negative impact to be produced, and educators should be wary of this.

- *Individual or collective:* IPE might focus on individual learning and assessment or collective learning through small groups of students collaborating.
- *Work/employment-based or college-based:* IPE can occur in the workplace informally or formally (or the two combined). College-based IPE does usually tend to include practice or work-based placements.
- *Shorter or longer:* IPE can be brief (in a meeting or over a lunch break), or could be extended and last anything from weeks to years.
- *Sooner or later:* IPE can be introduced at many different stages in qualifying/post-qualifying learning and subsequently at any stage throughout lifelong learning.
- *Common or comparative:* IPE can be concerned with learning needs across all the professions included or about respective roles, responsibilities, powers, duties and perspectives to inform collaboration in practice.
- *Interactive or didactic:* IPE tends to use small group, interactive methods where different professionals can interact, and didactic lecturing approaches tend to be used much less.

In practice, the form of IPE will be dependent not just on the aims of the programme, but also on availability of participants, funding and willingness of people to collaborate. As a result, IPE programmes are usually the result of a series of trade-offs and negotiations. For example, at pre-qualifying level the timing, length and focus of the programme will depend on when different groups of students can be freed from their core uniprofessional programme to be in the same place at the same time, and in a room that is sufficiently large to hold them all! Further, the methods of teaching and learning will depend on the numbers of students involved; small group, interactive learning is likely to require staff facilitators, and hence their availability is also an important determinant.

Particularly with longer courses, certain dimensions may be more – or less – appropriate at different points of the programme. Moreover, when designing IPE programmes it may seem obvious which of these forms are the most appropriate, and decisions relating to these dimensions might be made implicitly rather than as the result of an explicit discussion. However, there is much to be gained by making the pedagogical assumptions clear from the beginning, and being clear about how and where the learning outcomes are to be achieved. Also, if you go on to write a report or an evaluation of an IPE programme, it is very useful to describe which form the programme took so that readers can quickly gain a clear picture (Chapter 4 expands on the issue of evaluation in more detail). Box 1.4 gives an example of an evaluation of an IPE programme designed for professionals working in community mental health services and the dimensions it incorporated. We return to this particular example later in the book.

Box 1.4: The dimensions of a post-qualifying IPE programme for professionals working in community mental health services: an example

The Birmingham programme was *explicit* in its focus on learning to promote collaboration. It was *integrated* in that interprofessional education was a distinct emphasis reflected in the design, content and learning methods. Explicit teaching about interprofessional collaboration however comprised only *part* of the programme which also emphasised learning about psychosocial interventions and user participation. It was of course *particular* in its concern for people with severe mental health problems. The learning methods and assessments were generally *individual* rather than collective. Although all students were working in mental health services, the teaching programme was *college-based*, but with work-based assignments. It was a *long* course, lasting one day a week for two academic years and at a *later* stage of education; students had been qualified practitioners for at least two years. The curriculum contained both *common* elements, such as learning about psychosocial interventions and *comparative* study of respective roles and responsibilities and perspectives to inform interprofessional practice, especially in the modules on teamworking, inter-agency collaboration and assessment. These modules, especially, used *interactive* learning methods extensively, but others, for example a module on psychiatric symptoms and pharmacology were essentially *didactic*.

Source: Carpenter et al (2006, p 147; emphasis added)

Theoretical perspectives on IPE

The previous sections suggest that, in general, IPE has not always been clear about its precise aims, objectives, content and structure in terms of its different dimensions. However, there is a further aspect to IPE that has tended to be even less explicitly considered within the literature: links to underlying theory. As Barr (2002) notes, many reports on IPE are light on theory. Some commentators argue that without being underpinned by theoretical coherence in terms of choice of models, IPE will not be regarded as a substantive, informed practice (Craddock et al, 2006). A systematic review by Barr et al (2005) examined the extent to which the IPE literature is informed by theory in the description of method or in the choice of process or outcome measures. They found that only about a quarter of studies tended to do so. Those that were, primarily linked to adult learning theory, reflective practitioner theory and theories associated with social and psychological studies of teamwork and group behaviour (Parsell and Bligh, 1999), and these are expanded on in more detail in Chapter 4.

However, given that the history of IPE has tended to be located in practice, it may not be entirely surprising that it is not pervaded with academic theories. Indeed, for this reason some IPE practitioners may resist an attempt to over-theorise the field. But theory does have important implications. Whichever educational theory underpins an

IPE programme brings with it certain assumptions about learning processes, and particular aspects to be satisfied. We would argue that, without an explicit concept of underlying educational theory, this has the potential to reduce the effectiveness of individual IPE initiatives. Without due consideration of such theory initiatives are less likely to be well thought out and their effectiveness will be reduced. Moreover, without sufficiently incorporating educational theory, the legitimacy of IPE may be undermined.

Perhaps unsurprisingly, adult learning theory has tended to be the theory most commonly associated with IPE. After all, adults make up the student bodies of IPE programmes, and many health and social care education and training programmes are based on concepts of adult learning theory. This theory is also sometimes known as adrogogy – the art and science of helping adults learn (Knowles, 1990). Adult learning is quite a broad umbrella and incorporates a wide range of different approaches, some of which are more informed by empirical evidence than others. The underpinning notion of this approach is that adults are self-directed. Unlike children, adults bring a great deal of experience into the learning process which can be a rich source to draw on, but which also usually means that adults need to see the value in learning something before they will undertake to learn it. This clearly has important implications for the design of educational programmes. Chapter 4 outlines educational theories that IPE might draw on in more detail, so we do not explore these any further at this point. However, it is important to re-iterate at this early stage that when designing IPE programmes you should have a clear idea of the educational theory(ies) that are appropriate to your aims and objectives, and you should be explicit about this in setting out the features of that programme.

In this first chapter we have covered quite a lot of ground: from definitions, a potted history of IPE in England and internationally, and an outline of the different forms that IPE might take. This overview has been necessarily selective in its function as a brief introduction to a range of key issues surrounding IPE. The remainder of the book seeks to build on this initial grounding, revisiting these basic concepts and offering practical and accessible – yet relevant and robust – evidence about how IPE programmes can be initiated, run and evaluated.

Reflective exercises

1. Think of a time when you have undergone uniprofessional training or education. To what extent did this process prepare you to work with others from different professions? Did you hold stereotypes or preconceptions of other professions before your course, and did the programme challenge or reinforce these perceptions?

2. Why do you think the government sees IPE as being important for health and social care professionals? What are the potential gains that may be made? What do you think the main challenges might be? Compare your answers with those of a friend or colleague from a different background.

3. Think of a time when you may have undergone education or training that may broadly be described as IPE or MPE. What was the experience like? Did you enjoy it? Were there any particular difficulties or challenges that this experience raised?

4. Think about an IPE programme you have been on or read about. What were its aims and objectives? Which of Barr's dimensions of IPE (see Box 1.3) did this programme incorporate?

Further reading and resources

* Hugh Barr and his colleagues have produced a number of key introductory texts for IPE, including *Interprofessional education today, yesterday and tomorrow: A review* (2002) and *Effective interprofessional education* (Barr et al, 2005).

Relevant websites for official UK health and social care policy include:
* Department of Health: www.gov.uk/government/organisations/ department-of-health
* Department for Education: www.gov.uk/government/organisations/ department-for-education
* The Centre for the Advancement of Interprofessional Education (CAIPE), an independent charity that promotes and develops IPE as a way of improving collaboration between practitioners and organisations, engaged in both statutory and non-statutory public services. Their website hosts a range of supporting materials for individuals and organisations interested in IPE: www.caipe.org.uk/

Relevant websites for overseas organisations include:
* American Interprofessional Health Collaborative (AHIC): www.aihc-us.org/
* Australasian Interprofessional Practice & Education Network (AIPPEN): www.aippen.net/
* Canadian Interprofessional Health Collaborative (CIHC): www.cihc.ca/
* European Interprofessional Practice and Education Network (EIPEN): www.eipen.eu/
* Japan Interprofessional Working and Education Network (JIPWEN): http://jipwen.dept.showa.gunma-u.ac.jp/
* Nordic Interprofessional Network (NIPNET): http://nipnet.org/

In terms of the health and social care professions, relevant professional bodies include:

- Association of Directors of Adult Social Services (ADASS): www. adass.org.uk
- Association of Directors of Children's Services (ADCS): www.adcs. org.uk
- British Association/College of Occupational Therapists (COT): www. cot.org.uk
- British Association of Social Workers (BASW): www.basw.co.uk
- British Medical Association (BMA): www.bma.org.uk
- Chartered Society of Physiotherapy (CSP): www.csp.org.uk
- Nursing & Midwifery Council (NMC): www.nmc-uk.org
- Royal College of General Practitioners: www.rcgp.org.uk
- Royal College of Nursing: www.rcn.org.uk

2

What does research tell us?

As suggested in the previous chapter, IPE presently occupies a central role within the education and ongoing training of health and social care students and practitioners. Although there is a large and growing literature relating to IPE, it is somewhat limited in its nature. Much of the academic literature is based on descriptions of programmes and processes, with rather less consideration of the outcomes of IPE. Furthermore, there has been a tendency for research into the outcomes of IPE to be methodologically weak. As such, it is difficult to tell whether IPE 'works', not just in terms of its impact on participants, but particularly in terms of whether it makes any difference to the quality of care provided and improved outcomes for those who use services. This chapter is an attempt to move beyond descriptions of programmes, while acknowledging the importance and practicalities of advice relating to how to 'do' IPE. By drawing on a range of sources and case studies, the chapter aims to examine both the processes that make IPE effective, and the outcomes that it is thought to be able to deliver for service users.

Before moving on to consider these lessons in detail, it is perhaps first worth noting the nature of the IPE research evidence. Like most literatures, IPE has a positive slant in terms of reporting. That is, research and evaluations are much more likely to report positive than negative impacts, particularly in terms of entire programmes. However, some parts of the literature do flag up important areas where IPE has had negative impacts, and later in the chapter we offer an example of where this has happened. Often we can learn more from when programmes are not effective than where they have produced moderately positive impacts, and we would encourage practitioners to reflect on what did not work in addition to what did when reporting on IPE initiatives. For this revised edition of the book we have sought to include more international literature on IPE. This is helpful in the sense that it offers a greater breadth of evidence that we can draw on. However, the literature on policy transfer (see, for example, Dolowitz and Marsh, 2000; Benson and Jordan, 2011) reminds us that we should be wary of extracting lessons from one context and applying them in another. This is often of concern across international boundaries, but we should be equally wary of this across other forms of boundaries too. Furthermore, within the literature base there is much more research evidence for post-qualifying than pre-qualifying programmes. In the eight years since the first edition of this book this has not changed, and there is still relatively little on post-qualifying IPE. This chapter considers the evidence on post- and pre-registration in more detail, but it is worth illustrating this bias early on. When drawing on research evidence in formulating or delivering IPE it is important to bear in mind where the evidence came from and the circumstances surrounding it, as this may have important implications for evaluating the findings.

How can IPE be made more effective?

Effectiveness is a tricky concept. There are a number of parallels in debates about the effectiveness of collaboration and the effectiveness of IPE. The final book in this series (*Evaluating outcomes in health and social care*, by Helen Dickinson and Janine O'Flynn) deals with evaluating outcomes of health and social care collaboration in more detail (and Chapter 3 in this book deals with the evaluation of IPE in more depth), so we will not dwell on these issues here. Yet it is worth noting that a number of the debates in the two fields are quite similar. As suggested in the previous chapter, IPE initiatives may be conceived with different aims and objectives (just as health and social care collaborations often are). They may be underpinned by different educational theories and take a number of different forms (again, just like there are multiple theoretical drivers for collaboration). As such, there is no one template for IPE programmes and they will differ depending on a range of contextual factors. There is a large volume of descriptive literature that chronicles the processes of IPE and sets out what seems to work well in which circumstances, at least as far as what the participants think, and again, the collaboration literature also has a strong evidence base in terms of processes. However, both fields have been criticised for lacking rigorous evidence of effectiveness in terms of measurable outcomes (particularly for service users). Given that both collaboration and IPE have had such a wide range of potential benefits ascribed to them, any measure of effectiveness must relate to the purposes of the intervention. In other words, we must be clear about what it is that we wish to achieve by way of IPE, and then measure how well the intervention is achieving these aims.

Moreover, there is a further distinction we should make at this point – between the effectiveness of individual IPE interventions and of IPE as an overall approach, promoted as it is by government policy, conferences, journals and books such as this. The IPE 'movement' is often criticised for the lack of evidence of effectiveness, although this is not really fair because there is surprisingly little robust evidence about the effectiveness of UPE. The same situation applies to discussions of collaborative working – both have, to some degree, been recognised as being 'a good thing', which intuitively seems like they will have a positive impact without necessarily having evidence that unequivocally demonstrates this. But this tendency can easily lead to thinking about IPE as an end in itself, rather than as a means to an end. Unless the IPE movement is seen to deliver outcomes that are clearly underpinned by empirical data and theoretical models, it runs the risk of losing legitimacy and being seen as just another fad. In order for IPE to demonstrate that it is effective, Barr (2002, pp 33-4) suggests that it must:

- *Put service users at the centre:* involve service users and clients in designing, teaching, participating in and assessing programmes.
- *Promote collaboration:* apply learning to collaborative practice, collaboration within and between professions, within and between organisations and with communities, service users and their carers.
- *Reconcile competing objectives:* harmonise, so far as practicable, the aims and methods of IPE with those for MPE and UPE.

- *Reinforce collaborative competence:* reach beyond modification of attitudes and securing common knowledge bases to ensure competence for collaborative practice.
- *Relate collaboration in learning and practice within a coherent rationale:* give reasons why interprofessional learning improves interprofessional practice grounded in theory.
- *Incorporate interprofessional values:* be inclusive, equitable, egalitarian, open, humble, mutual, generous and reciprocal.
- *Complement common with comparative learning:* include comparative studies to facilitate learning from and about each other, to enhance understanding about respective roles and responsibilities and inform co-working.
- *Employ a repertoire of interactive learning methods:* avoid over-reliance on any one method.
- *Count towards qualifications:* assess IPE for awards to add value.
- *Evaluate programmes:* subject IPE to systematic approval, validation and research.
- *Disseminate findings:* inform other developments in IPE.

Although we would not argue against any of these laudable aims, there is an important question as to whether IPE can realistically achieve all of these. Again, it is important at this point to differentiate between IPE as a movement and individual IPE programmes. Clearly, not all individual IPE programmes will be able to achieve all these measures, but for the IPE movement as a whole, this may be more realistic. It is also worth reiterating at this point that UPE and training programmes have not been subject to the same degree of scrutiny as IPE. There is surprisingly little robust evidence about the outcomes of professional education published in the specialist journals about social work, medical and nursing education, a fact that is confirmed whenever researchers undertake systematic reviews of these fields. In their study of the value of leadership development programmes across a whole range of different industries, Peck and Dickinson (2010) found that there is relatively little evidence to demonstrate that these activities have any impact on the outcomes of organisations. Once again, there are plenty of accounts of educational practice and theory, but few studies of outcomes beyond the degree of satisfaction of those taking part. However, IPE generally has to fight for its place in the curriculum or in agency training plans. It is often seen as inconvenient, expensive and troublesome to organise. It is not surprising, therefore, that proponents of IPE are frequently asked to justify it, and to answer the question, does it work?

We think the question of effectiveness is quite fair to ask. But it is not a simple question. Coming back again to the issue of collaboration and its similarities with the field of IPE, both have gained such attention because they are intuitively seen as important and necessary mechanisms in improving public services in a range of ways. However, neither is the panacea to resolving all the issues in their respective fields, and both need to be treated in a more analytical and nuanced way than they have tended to be thus far. This is a key message of this text and one to which we will return again later.

As suggested in the previous section, there is a range of factors that have the potential to act as barriers or enablers of effective IPE. Oandasan and Reeves (2005) suggest that these can be subdivided into issues directly related to the learner, the teaching environment and the institutional environment. These can also be classified as the *micro level* (for example, socialisation processes), *meso level* (for example, administrative challenges for learners and teachers that affect the teaching environment and the role of local leaders) and *macro level* (for example, the need for senior management and government political support). These levels are interdependent in practice, and decisions and actions that take place at one will effect those at another. This chapter considers all three levels, as should anybody who is planning on instigating a programme of IPE. Although there will inevitably be trade-offs involved in any planning process, it is likely that designers of IPE programmes will have a significant influence over the micro and meso levels, but less so on the macro level. However, as previously suggested, by evaluating IPE programmes and making evidenced recommendations, there is the potential for designers and evaluators of single IPE programmes to feed into the IPE movement as a whole, which may in turn influence this macro (strategic) level.

A final point to note (and again there are similarities here with the literature on collaboration) is that IPE programmes may go through different stages over their life course. Things are tried and tested and then developed to see if they can be improved. Further, as we encounter changes in terms of the macro level either in terms of the policy context or technologies available, we may see programmes change their focus or develop in new ways. As an illustration of this we provide a summary of the interprofessional scheme at the University of the West of England (UWE), set out in Box 2.1.

Box 2.1: The evolution of the UWE programme

In 2000 a pre-qualifying interprofessional curriculum was implemented to provide an ongoing interprofessional experience, which was perceived to be a key element missing from the previous curricula. Professional pathways comprised uniprofessional, shared multiprofessional modules and a discrete interprofessional learning strand. Three compulsory, formally assessed interprofessional modules were designed for delivery in academic settings, with students taking one in each year of their study. These three modules adopted an evidence-based learning approach, with students working together in small interprofessional groups to achieve both broad subject-based learning outcomes and to acquire essential skills for teamwork and collaborative approaches to care. This was logistically challenging given that each year there were between 1,000 and 1,200 students.

Between 2000 and 2010 there were a number of relatively minor changes made to the content and delivery of the modules to improve their running and effectiveness. In 2010 there was a radical revision of the curriculum that saw the removal of the year 1 module and the redesign of courses in years 2 and 3. The year 1 module was removed in order to allow students to develop a fuller understanding of their own professional grouping before engaging with other professions. It was also felt that the introductory nature of this module was no longer necessary in the sense that the need for interprofessional working was a core consideration of all professional courses. The year 2 course was revised to be more challenging and also to recognise the importance of the central position of service users and carers and the involvement of wider agencies such as the police, child protection groups and third sector organisations. The year 3 course was changed although not as much as some would have liked. The idea was to focus the programme overall more toward being practice-facing, but to do this wholesale would have involved a significant change for mentors who have already recently experienced significant change. The module has kept the format of online delivery to facilitate small mixed student groups where students bring their experience from their practice settings to the module. Work is ongoing to establish whether it will be logistically possible to bring different groups of students together for learning opportunities when on placement, thereby having some interprofessional learning opportunities within practice.

Given such a broad student cohort, evaluations are mixed and some professions (for example, social work) have expressed concern about their ability to have their voices heard. One interesting observation has been that those students who have had the chance to develop a professional identity and a good understanding of their role have been better able to understand the relevance of interprofessional working and are more willing to participate actively. Online delivery is liked by some and not by others who have had technical difficulties or problems in accessing computer equipment.

A range of positive outcomes has been identified by students including their understanding of the need of interprofessional working, learning about self and communication confidence. A number also noted that it was not really until they moved to practice as a qualified professional that they fully realised the importance of pre-qualifying interprofessional learning. Despite the challenges, many of the staff reported enjoying the programme and learning through working with colleagues they may not ordinarily work with.

In terms of the future development of this programme of learning, a key challenge will be to examine how, and at what point, a service improvement focus and process can be incorporated into interprofessional learning.

This comes about in response to the macro context of fiscal constraint, and the need for health and social care organisations to make real and sustained cost efficiency savings.

Source: Adapted from an account by Pollard et al (2014, pp 75-83)

UPE, MPE or IPE?

As outlined in the previous chapter, although these terms have a tendency to be used interchangeably (particularly IPE and MPE), they are, in fact, quite different entities and are underpinned by different values and approaches. As also suggested, over the past 20 years or so the government has firmly reiterated the value of MPE and IPE, and it is generally expected that all health and social care pre-qualifying courses include interprofessional learning. Some commentators have suggested that this shift represents a sea change from traditional uniprofessional approaches to education where professions were educated as if in silos and never mixed. The inability to work with others was merely seen as a manifestation of this education process, which is a 'profound disconnect through which education is failing to adequately prepare students for their professional work' (Stumpf and Clark, 1999, p 30). However, it would be naive to assume that this signals the death knell for UPE. As we saw in the UWE case study in Box 2.1, the importance of UPE was confirmed through the introduction of a programme of IPE. All three approaches are important for learners for different purposes and at different points within learning careers. As such it is important that it is evidenced where and when these different approaches should be used and what differences they might make.

UPE is obviously crucial in imparting the specialised knowledge that professionals will need in order to carry out their roles successfully using specialised skills as required. But it does not necessarily follow that UPE cannot equip learners for working collaboratively with other professions. After all, collaboration – between professions and agencies – is not a new thing and has been taking place in practice with varying degrees of success for some time. As Miller et al (1999) suggest, UPE can do much to prepare learners for working with other professions. It is often suggested as the way in which learners are socialised into particular professions and assume, or reinforce, stereotypes about other professions. By exploring and challenging stereotypes through these channels learners may be better prepared for working in partnership. However, to our knowledge, there has not yet been a comparative study of the outcomes, in terms of attitudes, knowledge and skills in interprofessional working, of UPE versus IPE. It may well be, for example, that medical students would learn more about the roles of a social worker by receiving presentations from experienced social workers than by taking part in interactive workshops with social work students.

MPE is often regarded as a less effective way of preparing learners for collaboration, as there is limited formal contact between students. However, it can provide economies of scale. Essential common learning delivered via a didactic format to a large number of students can be much more efficient than delivering the same topic within uniprofessional settings. However, MPE on a large scale might potentially bring with it its own difficulties in terms of timetabling and accommodating large groups (see, for example, Tucker et al, 2003). Although the intention behind this mode of learning is not to improve collaboration between professions, learners will inevitably interact in an informal way in breaks or after teaching, or even during it if they are not particularly engaged! This interaction could possibly lead to students forming more positive views of other professions, although this cannot be presumed. For example, one group of students may believe that the lectures are being 'dumbed down' to accommodate the less academically able members of another group (thereby helping them feel superior, of course). Or they may think that the content is being slanted to meet the needs of another group of students. Drawing on contact theory (see Chapter 4 for more detail), Carpenter (1995a) found that even when interactions between different professions was positive, stereotypes still remained as individuals were not seen as 'representative' of their group. In other words, although learners had interacted positively with a group that they held negative stereotypes about, these were not broken down as they viewed the members of this group as somehow different to their peers.

It is important to remember that IPE will not be the most appropriate means of delivering all learning experiences. Most educators assume that IPE needs to involve small group work and significant interaction between learners. This is challenging in itself in terms of the delivery and facilitation of sessions, but there is also a range of other logistical problems that have to be overcome. Timetabling across departments and institutions can be a practical nightmare and joint accreditation and validation requirements can also be challenging. By comparison, UPE often looks quite simple. Box 2.2 illustrates a case study of an IPE training programme that, although evaluated positively by students, suffered from some such practical difficulties. Ladden et al (2006) suggest that some of these difficulties might be overcome by the use of electronic technologies. However, these cannot provide the face-to-face interaction that most people would consider essential to fostering positive changes in interprofessional understanding and respect. In short, when designing and delivering IPE you should be mindful of the potential complexities of organising that you may encounter.

Box 2.2: IPE and practical difficulties

Hylin et al (2007) report on a two-week pre-qualification IPE course that was run on a 'training ward' in Sweden. This gave medical, nursing, physiotherapy and occupational therapy students hands-on experience of running a ward and caring for the patients. The aims were to enhance the students' understanding of the roles of other professions and the importance of communication for teamwork and patient care. Based on the positive findings from a follow-up questionnaire two years later, the authors suggest that IPE at pre-qualification can provide lasting impressions that promote teamwork in students' future careers. However, they also reported that during its course the programme encountered a series of practical difficulties. As there was only a small number of occupational therapy and physiotherapy students, they were not always present at all sessions. Medical students also had to miss some sessions due to a clash with lectures. Other students (occupational therapists and nurses) felt that this was inappropriate and perceived that medical students were not interested in teamwork. As the course took place in a ward setting, physiotherapists and physicians felt that it catered more to the needs of nursing students than themselves. Furthermore, most of the facilitators that were constantly present were nurses, so some students felt that nursing was considered the most important profession. There were occupational therapy, physiotherapy and orthopaedic surgery facilitators attached to this course, but they tended to end up with other duties to attend to, which clearly sent out significant signals to the students.

When should IPE be delivered?

As suggested above, what it is that we are seeking to achieve with a learning experience and what resources are available will influence which form is most appropriate. Moreover, the point that learners are at in terms of their career is also an important factor in this decision. As suggested earlier, there is much more research relating to post-qualification IPE than there is relating to pre-qualification. This is somewhat of a challenge given that a recent review by Barr et al (2014) found that at least two-thirds of UK universities with qualifying courses in health and social care included IPE. IPE will never constitute the entirety of pre-qualification education and can only exist as one part of this, otherwise the need for a particular profession would be clearly undermined. Despite the spread of IPE into pre-qualification programmes in recent years there has been widespread debate over whether pre-qualification learners should be involved in IPE at all, as they may not have fully developed their professional identity and may not have sufficient experience to share. Studies have shown that as early in as two months of a programme students have been found to already have strong stereotypical notions of their intended professions, and have clear ideas about the social status of this in comparison to other professions (see Box 2.3 for an example of this). Consequently, some authors have advocated addressing stereotyping in the early stages of professional education (Clark, 1997; Barr, 2000). There is some evidence that stereotypes can be changed, at least in short programmes for students in the final stages of their courses (Carpenter, 1995a, 1995b; Carpenter and Hewstone, 1996). However, as we shall see below, the evidence is mixed, with one programme reporting negative changes (Tunstall-Pedoe et al, 2003). As outlined in the example in Box 2.1, other experiences demonstrate that if students have not had an opportunity to fully develop their professional identity, then a programme of IPE might not be as effective as it could be. Clearly there isn't one easy answer to the question of when IPE should come in terms of educational sequencing, and will need to remain under close consideration.

Box 2.3: Stereotyping by pre-qualification students

Lindqvist et al (2005) report on a pre-qualification interprofessional learning programme run by the Centre for Interprofessional Practice at the University of East Anglia. This involved first year students from six different health professions working together in small cross-professional groups discussing issues relating to interprofessional working. The main learning objectives of this initiative were to:

- identify key principles that facilitate successful interprofessional teamworking;
- reflect on why effective interprofessional practice is important to service users;
- reflect on their own role as health professionals, and begin to learn about the role of other healthcare professions;
- begin to understand the benefits of and constraints to good interprofessional teamworking.

At the outset of the programme students already had clear differences in attitudes that were measured using particular evaluation tools. They had clear views about which professions were the most caring and the least subservient. These views were measured at the start and end of the programme, and contrasted with those of a comparison group who had not received IPE. The researchers suggest that, 'the students in the intervention group tended to view the different health professionals as being more "caring" and less "subservient" at the end of the intervention' (Lindqvist et al, 2005, p 515).

Although this study was relatively small scale and the participants in the IPE were self-selecting and to some degree were probably more open to the influences of such a programme, these results do suggest some key lessons. First, learners have strong stereotypes of other professions early on within their educational careers, and second, IPE is able to influence the opinions and attitudes of students. Feedback from the students who took part in the initiative was positive, and consequently the university introduced IPE as a permanent part of the pre-qualification timetable.

Whether IPE is pre- or post-qualification also tends to influence where the learning will take place. Barr et al (2014) found, in a survey of pre-qualification IPE programmes in health and social care, 55% of courses were provided only in universities, 9% on placement, and 35% comprised a mix of placement and university. Post-qualification IPE is more likely to be work-based and pre-qualification university-based. From a review of the literature Barr (2000) suggests that work-based IPE is markedly more likely than university-based IPE to improve the quality of services and/or bring direct benefit to service users. Drawing on adult learning theory (see Chapter 4) this would seem to make sense, given that work-based learners will have real problems to overcome that may make learning more appealing and applicable to their everyday practice. Table 2.1 shows the various approaches that have been used in the UK at different stages of professional education, together with their primary learning outcomes. The examples chosen are all discussed elsewhere in this text. In some cases approaches are combined. For example, Morrison et al (2003) describe a programme for pre-qualifying medical and nursing students that began with two weeks of classroom–based learning followed by six weeks of shared placements on wards. They consider that learning in both contexts was effective when perspectives were shared, although while the classroom studies enabled the students to learn about teamwork, it was while on placement that they actually experienced what it felt like.

Table 2.1: Stage of education, methods of learning and teaching and intended outcomes

Stage of professional education	Methods of learning and teaching	Primary intended outcomes	Examples
Foundation (1st year)	Shared lectures and seminar groups Problem-based (or enquiry and action) learning (PBL/EAL) Joint community projects	Positive attitudes to other professions and to interprofessional teamworking and collaboration	Barrett et al (2003) Anderson et al (2006)
Advanced/specialist pre-qualifying (3rd/4th year)	Classroom-based PBL Clinical/practice placements Training wards Online PBL	Knowledge and skills about collaboration in relation to specialist concerns (eg ethics) and/ or user/patient groups	Morrison et al (2003) Reeves et al (2002)
Post-qualifying	External short courses and workshops	Improved knowledge and skills as above	Reeves and Sully (2007)
Post-qualifying	Team-based training in workplace	Team development/ quality enhancement	Reeves and Freeth (2006)
Post-qualifying/ postgraduate	University-based programmes and modules within programmes	Advanced knowledge and skills in specialist areas or methods	Carpenter et al (2006)

Planning and delivering IPE

Although IPE is often presented as being a new or different way of delivering education, in practice, designing and delivering a programme has much in common with the design and delivery of UPE or traditional training and education programmes. IPE will inevitably draw on theoretical and educational models that are appropriate to the specific settings and contexts it will encounter, but there are still many pertinent lessons that may be drawn from learning theory more widely. As such, although it is clearly important to consider the particular connotations that IPE brings with it, educators should not disregard all standard educational and learning theories, and there is much that can be drawn from these fields. As with any educational initiative, customary teaching procedures such as setting learning outcomes and objectives for programmes and sessions should be done as standard. In IPE planning is key and will be a major determinant of success. Being able to involve individuals who are enthusiastic and who have energy within this process will greatly increase an initiative's chances of overcoming what are often difficult obstacles in getting an IPE programme up and running.

Clearly the role of the teacher(s)/tutors is vital within any IPE programme. Ponzer et al (2004) concluded from their study of a training ward that the quality of clinical supervision was the most important contributor to the students' satisfaction. As previously indicated, adult learning theory is the most commonly cited basis for IPE programmes. Given this, teachers generally adopt the role of 'facilitator' (see, for example, Fox, 1994) or 'coach' (see, for example, Schön, 1987) within IPE programmes. Rather than simply teaching in a didactic sense, facilitators work with learners, generally with groups. As Barr (1996, p 244) stresses, the role of the facilitator is essential and this individual needs to be, 'attuned to the dynamics of interprofessional learning, skilled in optimising learning opportunities, valuing the distinct experience and expertise which each of the participating professions brings.' Hammick (1998) considers that facilitators who are successful in such roles are often those who are accustomed to interprofessional teamworking themselves and are able to deal with frictions that arise when different professions work together.

Thomas et al (2007) elicited the experiences of students and facilitators on a pre-qualifying IPE programme for nursing, therapy and social work students at UWE. The students worked in mixed groups of 12 for six two-hour sessions, in both their first and second years. Key findings from focus groups and interviews are presented in Box 2.4.

Box 2.4: Useful knowledge and skills for facilitators

- Facilitators greatly valued preparation sessions that the programme leaders had provided before the start of the programme and also peer support through facilitators' meetings in which they could share their experiences.
- In general, students preferred facilitators who were quite directive at the start and who provided guidelines and even structured exercises to get things going.
- Over time, the group would become less dependent and members would be able to use their own initiative to direct and support the function of the group. It is well to remember that the group is likely to demonstrate the familiar stages of group development ('forming, norming, storming and performing').
- An understanding of group dynamics was very important. Students appreciated facilitators who were flexible and knew when to draw in students who were in a minority (whether by profession, gender or ethnicity), when to offer a comment or information and when to stay silent. Conversely, facilitators could inhibit students' learning by controlling or rescuing the group so that they remained dependent.
- Facilitators can find it difficult to move students on from simply presenting the results of their enquiries to debating the issues involved. Effective techniques, included asking open questions, such as 'where does that leave us?' as well as specific invitations to comment, such as, 'what do other members think of the nurses' views on that?' Structured exercises such as role-play also proved useful in facilitating participation and debate.

Source: Adapted from Thomas et al (2007)

Another report from the UWE evaluation (Rees and Johnson, 2007) indicates that facilitating IPE groups was not for everyone. While many of the 28 facilitators who responded to a questionnaire survey enjoyed the experience, others found it stressful, even distressing. Facilitators concurred that it was an 'advanced skill' and not something that should be taken on lightly, especially by new and inexperienced staff.

The evidence from the UWE study emphasises the importance of groupwork skills in facilitating IPE groups, supporting Barr's (1996) assertion of their importance. But is Hammick (1998) also right in suggesting that facilitators need knowledge and practice experience in interprofessional working? At this point we do not really know. Thomas et al (2007) suggest that when the facilitators 'realised their role was to encourage students to look critically at the information students were presenting, they felt less anxious about their own lack of expert subject knowledge' (p 464). However, this conclusion needs to be tested out more widely, preferably through an independent external evaluation and with other student groups. For example, it is conceivable that students more used to a hierarchical style of teaching, learning and assessment (such as medical students) may be more concerned about the facilitator's perceived lack of expert knowledge. Similarly, professionals on a post-qualifying programme may need to feel quite confident that the IPE facilitators understand not only the roles and responsibilities of members of their own profession, but also those of other professions involved. Further, in an interprofessional context, students are much more attuned to partiality and will be understandably sensitive to any indications that their own profession is being presented unfavourably.

Although facilitators clearly have an important role to play in making IPE effective, the attitudes and roles that learners adopt will also have a significant impact on whether the initiative ultimately has any impact on these individuals and their activities. Barr (1998) outlines the knowledge, skills and attitudes that learners need to develop in order that professionals can work together more effectively (see Box 2.5). Arguably, some of these competencies will come to members of some professions more easily than others, and some will be more necessary within specific contexts than others. However, the objectives of IPE are usually more than imparting technical knowledge of how to undertake specific activities; they are about attempting to cultivate ways and means in which professionals might work together more effectively. To this end, IPE initiatives that aim to develop the types of skills and attributes outlined in Box 2.5 may find that they are more successful than those that do not (Chapter 4 goes on to consider different models of learning and the potential impacts of these on IPE initiatives).

Box 2.5: Collaborative capacities

- Describe your roles and responsibilities clearly to other professions.
- Recognise and observe the constraints of your role, responsibilities and competence, yet perceive needs in a wider framework.
- Recognise and respect the roles, responsibilities and competence of other professions in relation to your own.
- Work with other professions to effect change and resolve conflict in the provision of care and treatment.
- Work with others to assess, plan, provide and review care for individual service users.
- Tolerate differences, misunderstandings and shortcomings in other professions.
- Facilitate interprofessional case conferences, team meetings etc.
- Enter into interdependent relationships with other professions.

Source: Adapted from Barr (1998, p 181)

As we have previously suggested, in practice IPE is often inevitably a series of compromises. Although there is a wealth of guidance about best practice in IPE, in actuality it may not always be possible to design and deliver IPE along these lines. As O'Halloran et al (2006, p 26) outline, 'curriculum design is always a compromise between the "educational idea", the teaching and learning resources available and what will work in the local context.' In other words, it is a series of compromises between the different levels (micro, meso and macro) that influence the context, design and execution of a programme.

However, as a helpful overview, Nasmith and Oandasan (2003) have produced a planning guide for IPE initiatives (see Box 2.6) based on Kotter's (1995) analysis of leading change initiatives in business environments. This list of questions is intended to guide individuals through the change process that they may encounter when introducing IPE initiatives. Each question builds on what has gone before, therefore overlooking any one question can potentially lead to difficulties later on in the design process.

Box 2.6: Key issues in planning IPE initiatives

1. What are the external/internal drivers influencing the development of this programme?
2. Who are your potential partners?
3. What is the overall goal of this activity at the interprofessional and profession-specific levels, that is, attitudes, skill development, team building?
4. What are the opportunities within the current learning context?
   - Service user population
   - Practice site(s)
   - Learners in terms of disciplines and level of training
   - Timing (scheduling, length of programme)
5. What barriers/difficulties do you anticipate and how can you overcome them?
6. Who are the key players in designing this intervention?
   - How will you involve them?
   - What will be their roles and responsibilities?
   - How will you build group trust and cohesiveness?
   - How will you resolve conflict?
7. What are the specific objectives of this activity?
   - Content
   - Essential elements of interprofessionalism
8. What teaching methods and tools will you use to operationalise these objectives?
9. How will you evaluate the activity?

- Reactions/satisfaction
- Learning (knowledge–attitudes–skills)
- Results (impact)

10. How will you ensure the sustainability of this programme?

- Funding
- Challenging the culture

Source: Adapted from Nasmith and Oandasan (2003)

Later, in Chapter 4, we look at useful frameworks and concepts in the design and evaluation of IPE, in particular at social psychological understandings of IPE as being an intergroup encounter and the lessons that may be drawn from this for curriculum design. First, however, we consider answers to the question frequently asked by sceptical colleagues, 'but does it work?'

Does it work?

As suggested earlier, IPE has been fairly widely critiqued for not having unequivocally and empirically demonstrated that it produces significant outcomes. As Nickol (2015, p 1) describes, 'although recent years have seen remarkable advancement in IPE's scope and impact, many questions remain unanswered.' Sceptics often cite a large-scale international systematic review (Zwarenstein et al, 2000) because it found a dearth of rigorous evidence linking IPE and outcomes. However, the research team note that this lack of evidence does not necessarily mean that IPE is ineffective, or that there is evidence of ineffectiveness. What this means is that no one knows whether IPE is effective (or not) in achieving improved collaborative practice or health and social care outcomes. This review was conducted according to the Cochrane process that permits only controlled and time series studies. In fact, of the 1,042 IPE studies identified, only 89 were retained for further consideration, and none of these met the inclusion criteria. At the time the research team noted that 'the need for dependable evidence of the effects of IPE is now pressing' (Zwarenstein et al, 2000, p 2), and went on to stress the importance of rigorous evaluation of IPE programmes (there is more detail on how to evaluate IPE in the following chapter).

Observing that many of the excluded studies nevertheless had much to offer the evidence base for IPE, the research team subsequently carried out a much more inclusive review, identifying 353 studies published by 2003, and report their findings in detail in Barr et al (2005). The review focused on 107 'high-quality' studies, just over half of which were published in the US and a third in the UK. Over three-quarters concerned post-qualifying programmes, which were generally short training events or workshops or much longer university-based postgraduate programmes. Only one in five courses was pre-qualification, but, as the reviewers predicted, since the review took place there has been a substantial number of well-designed studies of pre-qualifying IPE arising from common learning initiatives and other significant publications are emerging (see, for example, Pollard et al, 2006).

The call for better methodological designs in the study of IPE was heeded to some degree in the sense that when the Cochrane review was updated in 2013 there were 15 quantitative studies, including eight RCTs, with sufficiently rigorous methodologies to merit their inclusion (Reeves et al, 2013). All of these studied the effectiveness of the IPE intervention in comparison to no educational intervention. Of these, seven found positive outcomes in terms of diabetes care; emergency department culture and patient satisfaction; collaborative team behaviour and reduction of clinical error rates for emergency department teams; collaborative behaviour in operating rooms; management of care delivered in cases of domestic violence; and mental health practitioner competencies related to the delivery of patient care. Four studies also found that IPE had no impact on either professional practice or patient care and a further four reported mixed outcomes. Again the authors noted that because of the small number of studies and their variation, it was difficult to find generaliseable inferences about the key elements of IPE and its effectiveness.

Barr et al (2005) attempt to unpack the concept of IPE and its impact by suggesting that, where done effectively, IPE can start a chain reaction that has an impact on individuals, organisational performance and service user care (see Figure 2.1). By creating trust between different professions, collaboration may be encouraged that will reduce stress on individuals, improve the team atmosphere, increase satisfaction, increase staff retention and improve quality of care through happier staff and greater collaboration (which will ultimately improve collaborative working). This is a fairly bold set of claims, particularly given concerns that collaborative working has not empirically demonstrated that it necessarily leads to better outcomes for service users. However, the team point out that 'examples of IPE, however carefully chosen, cannot establish conclusively each link in the above chain' (Barr et al, 2005, p 28). This is partly related to issues over the rigour of evaluation designs, but is also related to the ability to attribute changes in practice, and ultimately service user outcomes, to a programme of education. How is it possible that what can be a relatively small input in terms of teaching or education can be demonstrated to sustain changed practice and deliver outcomes in terms of individual job satisfaction, stress levels and the experiences of people who use services? Barr et al (2005) further note that IPE alone will not succeed in delivering all these changes, but must also be used in conjunction with different approaches in order to be effective.

What Figure 2.1 usefully illustrates is that the outcomes of IPE may take place at a range of different levels. When we think in terms of IPE and outcomes we are not simply thinking about whether the participants appreciated the experience and considered that they learned something about interprofessional working. Moreover, we are not just thinking about outcomes for service users, but there is a range of impacts at other levels that may be brought about by IPE, and that may also ultimately have an impact on the lives of service users in the longer term. In Chapter 4 we outline a framework that is often used within the IPE evaluation literature to categorise these outcomes, and we will say more then about a range of outcomes at these different levels.

Figure 2.1: IPE chain reaction

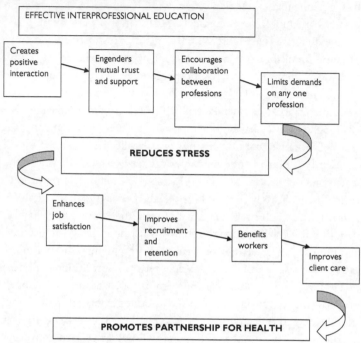

Source: Adapted from Barr et al (2005, p 27)

This chapter concludes by offering examples of some selected instances where IPE has demonstrated both positive and negative impacts.

Pollard and colleagues (2004, 2005, 2006) report a longitudinal evaluation of pre-qualifying IPE at UWE (described in Box 2.1). This tracked students from the beginning of their programmes of study and over the next three years using measures developed and validated for the study (see Chapter 4 for further details of these, and other validated outcome measures). The findings, which contain both positive and negative results, are summarised in Box 2.7.

Box 2.7: UWE evaluation of pre-qualifying IPE for health and social work

At UWE, each year of the pre-qualifying courses for nursing, social work, occupational therapy, radiotherapy and diagnostic imaging all contain an 'interprofessional module'. Learning takes place in small groups employing EAL, which, significantly, is assessed. In the third year, learning is online. Data are reported for around 500 students who completed the various scales at the three time points. In general, students at the beginning of the programme were positive about IPE and about their own communication and teamwork skills, but neutral in their views about interprofessional interaction. However, in their second year they became less positive about IPE, communication and teamwork skills, and negative about interprofessional interaction. Pollard et al (2005) termed this 'second year scepticism'. In the third year, their self-ratings of communication and teamwork skills returned to first year levels, but there was no further change in attitudes to IPE, and they became even more negative about interprofessional interaction – hardly the result that the programme hoped for.

The temporary reduction in self-ratings of communication and teamwork may be understood in terms of a drop in confidence from unrealistically high initial ratings (you don't know how much you don't know until you start learning). Again, as the researchers suggest, attitudes to IPE at the start may also have been idealistic. Nevertheless, at the end of the programme, around 70% of the participants were still positive about IPE and only about 10% actually negative. In contrast, the startling finding was that at qualification hardly any of the participants gave positive ratings about interprofessional interaction; the proportions of negative responses ranged from 46% for adult nursing students to 95% for social work students. Why should this be so?

One interesting observation is that older and more experienced students entered the programmes with more negative views of interprofessional interaction than younger and less experienced students. Perhaps these students 'contaminated' the learning groups with their negative views? The researchers consider that this was not the case because these students' comparatively negative views had not been maintained in the second year. Alternatively, it may be that IPE, as the researchers suggest, raises awareness of the problems and inequalities that impede interprofessional collaboration. The increased proportion of negative views in the third year may largely reflect students' experiences on practice placements. The Interprofessional Interaction Scale (IIS) used in this study is probably tapping perceptions of the world of interprofessional collaboration as it is: professionals have stereotyped views of each other; there is a status hierarchy; and professionals do not always communicate or cooperate. In other words, the students may simply be being more realistic. In that case, these should not be construed as 'negative' findings.

Mixed findings about the outcomes of pre-qualifying IPE were also reported by Tunstall-Pedoe et al (2003) who evaluated a 10-week 'common foundation programme' in the first term for medical, allied health and nursing students at St George's Medical School and Kingston University in London. Instead of a hoped-for reduction in negative stereotypes, the researchers found that at the end of the programme stereotypes had actually worsened. For example, doctors were viewed as significantly less caring, less dedicated, more arrogant, and less good communicators and team players than at the start. Similarly, nurses were considered less dedicated, more detached, less hard-working and not such good communicators. There were statistically significant reductions in the proportions of students giving positive ratings about IPE, such as whether or not it enhanced their own learning. Nevertheless, almost all who responded at the end of the programme still believed that IPE would enhance interprofessional working and lead to better service user care.

Zwarenstein et al (2005) found that there is a growing body of research that shows the positive effects of post-qualifying IPE on the delivery of care, although this is patchy and often weak in primary care settings. The research team outline positive impacts on the delivery of care in a range of areas including geriatric evaluation and management, congestive heart failure, neonatal care and screening. Positive impacts were reported for a wide range of groups, from children to older people and individuals with sexually transmitted infections. Box 2.8 illustrates some programmes that have reported positive impacts of IPE.

Box 2.8: Positive impacts of IPE

The examples cited here are just a small proportion of a number of studies that have outlined various impacts that IPE may have on a range of different forms of outcomes.

A short (four-session) course in 'teamworking and family conferencing' in palliative care was designed for groups of medical and social work students (10 of each) in a university medical centre in the US. Students took part in case discussion and role-plays, shared personal experiences of death and dying, and visited a service user and family in the centre. The course was evaluated by Fineberg et al (2004) using a quasi-experimental design in which changes in their knowledge and understanding of roles and responsibilities were compared to a group of students who had volunteered to participate in the course, but who had been unable to do so for practical, timetabling reasons. These students were given the course reading only. Students who took the course reported statistically significant increases in knowledge, which was sustained at follow-up three months later. By contrast there were no significant changes in the comparison group.

Reeves and Sully (2007) report on a UK university-based IPE initiative concerning services for victims and survivors of intentional and unintentional violence. The course was designed to enable practitioners from a range of statutory sector bodies to work together along with colleagues from the voluntary and academic sectors to deliver expert services to a diverse range of service users. Results from the evaluation found that participants changed some long-held negative stereotypes about colleagues working in different professions and agencies. The course also enhanced the knowledge of learners and their working relations with different staff. Furthermore, some learners suggested that it had improved their confidence to work on an interprofessional basis and had led to changes in their organisation's practices.

Rogowski et al (2001) report on how IPE was used within the context of a quality improvement programme across 10 self-selecting neonatal intensive care units in the US. The very low weight infants who were treated on these wards were relatively high-cost per service user. The multidisciplinary teams received instruction on quality improvement and undertook a series of improvement initiatives. Over the three-year study period significant cost savings were made (US$2.3 million across the sites after the first year alone), while costs in the control group rose over the same period. Moreover, these cost savings appeared to be sustainable and quickly offset the institutional expenditure for quality improvement efforts.

The MedTeam's project (Morey et al, 2002) was a team training intervention for doctors and nurses developed from one used with aircrew that had been shown to reduce 'aviation mishaps'. The project's aims were to reduce the number of similar 'adverse incidents' in emergency departments in selected US hospitals. The curriculum focused on communication, problem solving, resources and workload management. Teaching methods included presentations and practical exercises concerning real-life tasks. Team performance was rated by trained observers and was judged to have improved significantly compared to the comparator teams that did not receive the intervention. Furthermore, the 'clinical error' rate reduced from 30% to only 4%.

A similar training intervention, also in the US, was designed to improve teamworking in stroke rehabilitation units (Strasser, 2008). This involved practitioners from medicine, nursing, occupational therapy, speech language pathology, physiotherapy and social work. The six-month programme included an interactive workshop on team dynamics, problem solving, using performance feedback and developing action plans for process improvement. This was followed up with telephone and video conference consultations. Outcomes for over 500 patients of 14 teams that received the intervention were compared to a control group from 13 teams. There was a statistically and clinically significant improvement in motor functioning in the intervention group compared to the controls.

However, there were no differences in the mean length of stay, which is likely to be affected by organisational factors as well as patient functioning.

The University of Birmingham programme on interprofessional community mental health (see Box 3.3 later for further details) included training in psychosocial interventions, such as cognitive behaviour therapy and family therapy, as well as user-centred and interprofessional teamworking. Outcomes for service users with whom the students worked were assessed over six months using a number of validated measures of mental health and social functioning (which includes personal relationships and 'life skills'). There was no change in mental health status, but strong statistical evidence of improvement on the measure of social functioning. When compared to the outcomes for equivalent groups of service users in two other districts where the professionals had not been trained, it was evident that the service users had improved significantly more than the comparison group (Carpenter et al, 2006).

Reflective exercises

1. Think of an educational or training experience you have had and that you think was particularly *effective*. What made you think this was effective? What were the key factors that contributed towards this effectiveness?

2. Think of an educational or training experience you have had and that you think was particularly *ineffective*. What made you think this was ineffective? What were the key factors that contributed towards this ineffectiveness?

3. What are the specific circumstances in which you think that UPE and MPE would be appropriate in your field of work or study? If there are circumstances when more than one form would be appropriate, which would you choose, and why?

4. Draw up a list of the possible pros and cons of IPE for first year pre-qualification students. What more evidence would you need to decide on the optimal time for introducing IPE?

Further reading and resources

There have been a number of reviews of IPE that provide useful summaries of the literature. Additionally, there are also a number of commentaries based on these reviews. For further details, see:

- Barr et al's 'Evaluating interprofessional education' (1999), *Evaluating interprofessional education* (2000), *Effective interprofessional education* (2005) and *Interprofessional education* (Barr, 2015).
- Zwarenstein et al's *Interprofessional education* (2000), 'Effectiveness of pre-licensure interprofessional education and post-licensure collaborative interventions' (2005) and 'Interprofessional collaboration' (2009).
- Freeth et al's *A critical review of evaluations of interprofessional education* (2002) and *Effective interprofessional education* (2005a).
- Institute of Medicine's (US) *Measuring the impact of interprofessional education on collaborative practice and patient outcomes* (2015).
- Thistlethwaite's 'Interprofessional education' (2012).
- The *Journal of Interprofessional Care* is published six times a year and primarily aims to promote collaboration within and between education, practice and research in health and social care, and is a useful source of case studies and important lessons for individuals and organisations seeking to initiate, establish and evaluate IPE programmes: www.tandf.co.uk/journals/titles/13561820.html
- The *Journal of Research in Interprofessional Practice and Education* (JRIPE) is an open access North American online journal that disseminates theoretical perspectives, methodologies and evidence-based knowledge to inform interprofessional practice, education and research to improve healthcare delivery, quality of care and health status for individuals, families, and communities: www.jripe.org/index.php/journal

- The *Journal of Interprofessional Education & Practice* is a new quarterly online-only subscription journal affiliated with the University of Nebraska Medical Center, USA. It aims to provides innovative ideas for interprofessional educators and practitioners through peer-reviewed articles and reports: www.journals.elsevier.com/journal-of-interprofessional-education-and-practice/

3

Hot topics and emerging issues

Having explored key concepts and summarised key findings from the research, this chapter examines three key issues concerning IPE in health and social care settings. These hot topics were chosen because they are the ones about which we are asked most:

- How can we involve service users and carers within the process of IPE? Does this make any difference to outcomes for trainees and, ultimately, for people who use services themselves?
- How can we 'mainstream' and sustain IPE in education and training for health and social care?
- How can IPE programmes be effectively evaluated?

Involving service users in IPE

A key theme of health and social care policy concerns enabling service users (patients/clients) and carers to take a more central and active role in the organisation and delivery of their care. This policy has been extended to education to the extent that the DH (2002b) required social work education to involve service users and carers in the design and delivery of programmes. The General Medical Council (GMC) set out similar requirements in 2009 followed by the Health and Care Professions Council (HCPC) which regulates educational standards for allied health professionals and social care (2014).

There are a variety of ways in which service users may be involved in IPE. The earliest examples in the literature describe service users or carers sharing their experiences with mixed groups of professionals, either through presentations ('testimonials') or by allowing themselves to be interviewed by the students. For example, Turner et al (2000) describe a series of palliative care workshops during which medical, nursing, social work and rehabilitation therapy students interviewed the family carers of people with a terminal illness. The students were given instructions to find out which professionals were involved with the family, and to explore how the professionals had, or had not, collaborated effectively. As is common in such cases, the students reported in feedback interviews that they found the experience of meeting carers (or service users) profound and moving, and they considered that it would have a significant effect on their future practice as professionals. The carers likewise found the experience very positive, although it was evidently emotionally demanding, and this raises a question about the sustainability and acceptability of such initiatives. Is it fair to ask service users and carers to repeatedly lay themselves emotionally bare in the interests of professional education? Training based on personal history and insight is relatively new, and there is little evidence about its effects on service users and carers (see also Daykin et al, 2002). Levin (2004) offers guidance in the context of social work education, but this is also clearly relevant to IPE. The key steps are summarised in Box 3.1 (for guidelines concerning the involvement of mental health service users, see Tew et al, 2004).

Why an IPE programme is seeking to involve service users and at what level will determine how and when service users should be involved within processes of planning, delivery and evaluation. These factors will have an impact on the amount of training, support and input service users will need throughout these processes. Trainers and facilitators may likewise need support to understand what to expect, the types of questions that should and should not be asked in educational settings and how to support service users.

There is a range of reasons why service users might want to become involved with IPE programmes. Some may have an interest in teaching, but others may not. As such, the types of training offered will need to be varied and flexible. Some training may simply equip service users to be able to make the most of their contribution to a programme for themselves and for the learners involved. Others may wish to use the opportunity as a springboard to other educational opportunities. Particularly within academic settings it may therefore be possible to involve service users within training courses that may lead to a recognised teaching qualification or to act as foundation experience for a degree course. There are also a range of voluntary and community sector organisations around the country (many of which are service user-led) that may be able to offer this specialised training for both service users and educators. Whatever option is chosen, the important issue here is that both service users and educators are offered training and support so that they may both be more effective in their engagement in the process and get back what it is they want from this involvement without undue negative experiences.

We should not expect service users to be involved in what will often be a challenging process without payment, although this can be problematic. This can become particularly pernicious when the service user is in receipt of benefits that will be subject to rules about how many hours they may work and the level of income they may receive. There are no set rates for service user involvement in IPE and the amount available can vary substantially. They may be offered a visiting lecturer rate, or, if paid through a service user group, may charge a flat rate per day. Others may be paid in kind through access to facilities or services, while others may yet prefer to offer their work as a public service. But if service users are not to be paid at the same – or a similar rate – to other partners, it may send out a clear symbolic message. Further, it is good practice to always make sure that the programme covers any out-of-pocket expenses (including preparation costs, telephone calls, photocopying etc). It is important at the outset, therefore, to have a clear and frank discussion about expectations and remuneration to ensure that all stakeholders are happy with the arrangement. There are a number of guides available that deal with the issue in much more detail than we have done here (see, for example, Scott, 2003; DH, 2006).

As a first stage in planning any programme of IPE it is essential that stakeholders consider the appropriateness of service user and carer involvement and the extent to which they might be engaged in its planning and delivery. IPE programmes should be clear about this from the start, in terms of levels of involvement and the reasons for this with all stakeholders. This should allow service users to make informed decisions about their involvement. But first, as we have been emphasising throughout this book, everyone should know what the programme is aiming to achieve.

There are a number of reasons why service users and carers might be involved in IPE. At a basic level, they may be a good source of information so that students may be able to better understand what the issues they are discussing really 'feel' like. They may reflect the complexity of the system of care they are involved with and provide a different perspective. As such, service users may be involved as teachers – making presentations and facilitating – or co-facilitating in small groups. For example, Cooper and Spencer-Dawe (2006) describe how, at the University of Liverpool, trained service users were employed in a pre-qualifying IPE programme as co-facilitators in workshop sessions, and a service user, a student and a clinician were involved in the delivery of a pre-workshop plenary. Cooper and Spencer-Dawe provide a helpful account of the steps they took to develop the programme, which are very much in accord with Levin's guidelines (Box 3.1), and they include details of the accredited training programme undertaken by service user-trainers. An interview-based evaluation of the Liverpool programme compared the perspectives of students who had taken part in groups co-facilitated by service users to those led by staff alone. The authors concluded that there was some evidence that 'the number of hours contact with service users therefore appeared to be associated with an increased awareness that patients should be at the centre of the interprofessional team care process' (Cooper and Spencer-Dawe, 2006, p 300).

Box 3.1: Practical steps to involving service users in IPE

Step 1: Secure resources
- Allocate a budget to pay service users for their participation in the development of the programme as well as for any teaching that they will do. Ring-fence time for the staff involved.

Step 2: Decide who will lead on service user involvement
- Setting up and sustaining service user involvement requires a lot of time, skill, determination and effort. It also needs a lead (or leads) who will take responsibility.

Step 3: Define who service users and carers are
- Service users are sometimes called 'experts by experience'. What kinds of expertise and experience do you want them to have? It may be helpful to develop a person specification to help recruit the people you need.

Step 4: Set the level of involvement from the outset
- Be very clear about the principles, aims and intended outcomes of service user involvement, and agree this with prospective partners. Failure to do so can result in disillusioned service users who are understandably unwilling to participate.

Step 5: Provide training and support
- The kind and level of training service users may need will differ according to the nature of their participation. For example, service users who are designing and delivering a course module may benefit from a course on teaching adults. Effective support may include de-briefing after giving a presentation and/or peer support groups.

Step 6: Pay service users for their involvement
- Payment is often complicated and can affect the benefits service users receive. The fee should include travel expenses, telephone calls and allowances for personal assistants and replacement care. Make sure they can get the money quickly.

Source: Adapted from Levin (2004)

Beyond largely uncritical descriptive accounts, there is very little robust evidence of the impact of involving service users and carers in IPE and healthcare education in general (Morgan and Jones, 2009). Nevertheless, we see service user and carer involvement in the delivery of their health and social care services as an ethical issue, grounded in principles of autonomy and informed choice. Moreover, service users should be able to drive the education of future health and social care professionals. If they really are to be at the centre of the delivery of health and social care services, then they need to be involved not only in delivering some aspects of education, but also in its planning and evaluation. Perhaps the most thorough example of such involvement reported in the literature was a two-year, part-time post-qualifying IPE programme run at the University of Birmingham, from 1997 to 2003. As Barnes et al (2000a) describe, service users were involved from the very beginning as members of the commissioning panel for the programme and its evaluation. They also participated as members of the programme management team and the advisory group for the external evaluation, as well in teaching. They even participated, following training, in the formal academic assessment of the students' practice-based portfolios, a process described by Bailey (2005). Bailey considers that the service users were able to provide detailed constructive, meaningful feedback on issues of real importance. Overall, Barnes et al (2000a, p 199) note that 'the involvement of users as stakeholders in a partnership created a "saliency effect" on the other partners so that, whether they were professional managers, educators or evaluators, their orientations accommodated a service user-perspective on their tasks.'

But what kinds of impacts might we expect from involving service users and carers in IPE? Just as we cautioned in the introductory text (see Glasby and Dickinson, 2014b) against the assumption that 'collaboration' is inevitably a 'good thing', so, too, must we examine the same assumption about partnerships with service users in IPE. As Towle (2007, p 1) suggests, 'if the inclusion of patients as active participants in education is to be more than a passing fashion, evidence will be needed to demonstrate that there are benefits to be had for learners, professional educators and patients alike, and that there is a connection between these benefits and improved outcomes.' Clearly, not all partnerships with service users will deliver all of these benefits. So what sorts of benefits might we expect? Wykurz and Kelly (2002) suggest a number of impacts for students, service users and carers and staff of involvement in professional education (both UPE and IPE). These are summarised in Box 3.2. The reports cited above by Turner et al (2000) and Cooper and Spencer-Dawe (2006) provide evidence from interviews and focus groups with members of all three groups of some of these positive impacts, and a further report from the external evaluation of the University of Birmingham post-qualifying programme by Barnes et al (2006) provides comprehensive information on the impact of service user involvement at a number of different levels. These are summarised in Box 3.3.

Box 3.2: Potential impacts of service user involvement in IPE

For learners
- Enables access to personal knowledge and experience of condition and use of services
- Deepens understanding
- Provides constructive feedback
- Reduces anxiety
- Increases confidence
- Influences attitudes and behaviour
- Improves acquisition of skills
- Increases respect for service users
- Places learning in context

For service users
- Uses their experience positively
- Uses their knowledge positively
- Acknowledges their expertise
- Creates a sense of empowerment
- Provides an opportunity to help future service users

- Increases their knowledge
- Provides new insights
- Improves their understanding of professionals

For trainers
- Provides additional teaching resources
- Improves quality of teaching
- Offers alternative teaching opportunities
- Develops mutual understanding
- Enlists new advocates
- Provides value for money

Source: Adapted from Wykurz and Kelly (2002, p 820)

Box 3.3: Outcomes of partnership with service users in the University of Birmingham post-qualifying programme in community mental health

This programme (as described in Box 1.4) had as one if its aims to increase awareness of the importance of working from a service user's perspective. Central to the programme was a strong value base that emphasised partnership working between service users and professionals in the development of user-centred care. The service users' most influential role was in teaching specialist modules, initially on a sessional basis, but later the University of Birmingham appointed two service users to the staff team as part-time lecturers. They also provided support to service users contributing to and participating in the programme as students.

The external evaluators collected and analysed data from observation, interviews with students and their managers, self-completion questionnaires, standardised measures of service users' mental health and quality of life, and service users' opinions of the quality of care they received. The last two components were evaluated in relation to outcomes for two comparison groups of service users in areas where no training had taken place. Key findings were:

- Reaction to service users as trainers was mixed. Many students valued hearing first-hand experiences, but some felt that they could not criticise service users' views in the way they might challenge professionals; they were afraid to ask questions fearing that they might say the 'wrong thing'. They were also critical of the teaching skills of some service users.
- Nevertheless, there were significant increases in students' self-reported changes in their attitudes, knowledge and skills about partnership with service users. Students and team managers cited numerous examples of changes in individual and team practice that they attributed to the programme.
- Overall improvement in the service users' social functioning was significantly greater than for those in the comparison group, although there were no significant differences in improvements in mental health status or life satisfaction.
- The service users were positive about the quality of care which they received, somewhat more so than the comparator groups.

Source: Reported in Barnes et al (2006)

Barnes and her colleagues concluded that the success achieved must in part be attributed to the original design of the Birmingham programme and the responsiveness of its staff. If service users are to be empowered in contributing to IPE, they cannot be expected simply to react to the status quo; their role is to influence change and those changes are likely to be in the programme itself as well as through the learning experiences of students.

Barriers and facilitators of mainstreaming and sustaining IPE

In Chapter 2 we cited Oandasan and Reeves (2005) who suggest that barriers and facilitators can be classified as the micro level (for example, socialisation processes), meso level (for example, administrative challenges for learners and teachers that affect the teaching environment and the role of local leaders) and macro level (for example, the need for senior management and government political support). As observed in Chapter 1, at the macro level, central government has been quite explicit about its commitment to IPE. To this extent it could be argued that there has been some structural commitment to IPE. However, the degree to which this has changed activities at an organisational level, and how far this has served to change attitudes towards IPE, is perhaps questionable. Again, there are parallels with the collaboration field here. Although a number of legal and structural technical 'fixes' have been achieved by central government, at the local level partners have often struggled with the issue of how to work together, and central government has remained relatively silent on this issue. There is a risk that if collaborations are not seen to have delivered, others will not wish to engage with this agenda. A number of authors have echoed similar fears in relation to IPE. Without demonstrating that IPE can produce outcomes that are verifiable by empirical data and without demonstrating that it is underpinned by robust theory, then, some commentators have suggested, IPE may be nothing more than a passing fad (see, for example, Barr, 2000; Craddock et al, 2006).

IPE has been high on the agenda of many local organisations as a result of recommendations made by successive reports that have followed critical incidents (see, for example, Secretary of State for Health, 2001; Laming, 2003). In other words, IPE is being pushed in a top-down manner. Moreover, organisations like CAIPE and initiatives such as CIPW are advocating best practice on behalf of IPE, trying to produce and support enthusiasm for IPE in a bottom-up manner. Yet despite this, the spread of high-quality IPE and interest in this field around the country remains patchy. Local programmes still find themselves coming up against very real barriers, which Meads (2007) suggests is largely the result of what he terms 'culture'. Lawlis et al (2014) undertook a comprehensive review of the literature into the barriers and enablers of embedding IPE into curricula of universities (HEIs). They identified 1,570 articles that spoke about barriers and enablers, and the key points are summarised in Table 3.1. The interesting thing about these factors is that eight have been identified as barriers and enablers in different studies, suggesting that what can be helpful in one context might hinder in another. The researchers conclude that there are five key fundamental elements that inhibit or enhance IPE success and/or sustainability:

- Government funding
- HEI funding
- Faculty development programme
- HEI institutional structures to support the embedding of IPE into health professional curricula
- Staff ownership and commitment across all disciplines involved in IPE programmes.

However, given the nature of the evidence base, 'without further research it is not possible to determine if all five fundamental elements are critical for enduring pedagogical change' (Lawlis et al, 2014, p 309), and further research is required into these factors.

IPE has often existed as an adjunct – or an add-on – to existing education programmes. If IPE is to be sustainable, and if the learning produced by IPE is to be sustained, then it must be 'mainstreamed' in educational terms. However, this is more than about integrating IPE into education's organisational, theoretical, financial or regulatory systems; IPE must be seen as culturally efficacious in the eyes of health, social care and education organisations. Barr and Ross (2006, p 103) illustrate this issue graphically:

> ... if "mainstreaming" is to be more than mere rhetoric IPE must pervade the culture of professional education, supported unequivocally by top management, backed by the spectrum of stakeholders, benefiting from core educational funding, owned equally by each of the constituent professional programmes, permeating uniprofessional and multiprofessional teaching and learning throughout. Easily said, less easily done!

Table 3.1: Embedding IPE in HEI: barriers and enablers

Level	Barriers	Enablers
Government and professional	Lack/limited financial resources Changes within the organisations and HEIs involved	Establishment of collaborative groups from different HEIs and organisations Stakeholder commitment Shared ownership and unified goals Government funding
Institution	Lack/limited financial resources Lack/limited support Limited faculty development initiatives Scheduling of IPE within current programme Health professional degree calendars – different lengths of degree year Different degree timetables Rigid/condensed curriculum Extra-curricula versus required course/unit Differences in assessment requirements	Funding by institutions Organisational structures within HEIs developed Faculty development programmes
Individual	Faculty attitudes Lack of reward for faculty High workload (including teaching and administrative) Lack/limited knowledge about other health professions Not understanding IPE concept Lack of perceived value Different student learning styles 'Turf' or professional battles Bias towards own profession Lack of respect towards other health profession/als	Skill of facilitator Enthusiasm of facilitator/staff Staff as role models Champions Understanding of IPE Shared interprofessional vision Showing of equal status regardless of position or background

Source: Adapted from Lawlis et al (2014, pp 307-8)

The task of sustaining IPE and implementing its learning in practice is far from straightforward, as Barr and Ross rightly observe. As suggested above, one of the ways in which we might start to change attitudes towards IPE and make it more culturally acceptable is through rigorous evaluation, and the final sector in this chapter deals with this issue in detail. At the micro level of the programme within an institution, sustainability is likely to depend significantly on the enthusiasm, dedication and personal effectiveness of key staff, and the extent to which their managers back them. These key staff will necessarily represent at least some of the professional groups involved in the programme; in a real sense, they should be a model of collaborative working. Again, we return to the similarity of themes within the literature between IPE and collaborative working more broadly. As suggested by Glasby and Dickinson in this series (2014b), collaboration tends to be more effective where it has key 'champions', at least initially, to get it off the ground. What is clear is that those involved need time, not just to develop the programme, but to monitor how it is working, to support the facilitators and to sort out problems as they arise. Promoting the successes of the programme, both within the institution and outside, is undoubtedly very important. This creates a positive aura around the programme and encourages favourable expectations in staff and students, including those yet to participate. For example, Spry (2006) has written an enthusiastic editorial in the student issue of the *British Medical Journal* endorsing the common foundation programme at St George's Hospital Medical School. Further, an 'external institutional review' by the QAA in 2005 featured the common foundation programme as an example of 'good practice'. Such positive feedback should certainly sustain the programme. Similarly, individual staff may be rewarded for their efforts and the status of IPE enhanced.

More effective evaluation

We suggested earlier that it is imperative that IPE is rigorously and appropriately evaluated in order to clearly demonstrate the processes that underpin effective IPE and the longer-term outcomes that may result. The evidence-based practice movement has gained great momentum within the UK (see Dickinson and O'Flynn, 2016), and without solid evidence underpinning IPE there is a risk that it will lose credence (Humphris and Hean, 2004). The major deficiencies in reports of IPE evaluation are:

- lack of information about methodologies and limitations;
- lack of information about the intervention itself (student numbers, duration, dimensions);
- inability to convincingly demonstrate cause and effect;
- no comparison between the effectiveness of IPE and UPE;
- uncertainty of the longer-term effectiveness (or otherwise) of IPE.

This section considers these factors in more detail, before going on to suggest a series of guidelines for IPE evaluation.

In the discussion of outcomes in Chapter 2 we mentioned the original Cochrane systematic review of IPE (Zwarenstein et al, 2000) that found no studies meeting its tight inclusion criteria, and the most recent only identified 15 (Reeves et al, 2013). Those identified lacked control groups or used unvalidated outcome measures. What these, and other systematic reviews make apparent, is that evaluating IPE is not easy (Freeth et al, 2002). IPE is thought to be able to produce outcomes at a number of different levels but often in terms of intangible or imperceptible changes to anyone but the individual learners. Changes sought are often in terms of values, beliefs and perceptions, and as such are not easily and readily measurable. The evaluations that these types of systematic reviews are looking to incorporate are essentially 'gold standard' trials – randomised controlled trials (RCTs) – controlled before-and-after studies or interrupted time series studies. However, these types of studies of educational initiatives are not always possible, and, in the case of RCTs, potentially unethical (imagine trying to randomly assign students to a no-education condition).

As a result, IPE research has predominantly taken the form of uncontrolled before-and-after studies, typically examining changes in attitudes, knowledge and skills as a result of the intervention (see, for example, Parsell et al, 1998). These kinds of approaches are generally seen as producing 'hard' evidence, but they assume that we can measure the changes that are taking place (that is, that we can quantify changes in attitudes, knowledge and skills). Furthermore, they generally only measure the impacts that are expected, and not any unanticipated impacts. As we have argued, it is also important to consider the processes of intergroup student interaction that go on within a programme. Qualitative approaches (based on participant observation, interviews, focus groups and so forth) offer a chance to consider such issues in further detail, but here there may be concerns about the reliability of the sampling and of the data, particularly if the evaluation is done internally by those responsible for the course; 'socially desirable' responses are more likely in these circumstances. In other words, when students are asked whether they think the approaches are useful and successful they may answer 'yes' simply because they are being asked by the person who delivered the session or programme, rather than because this is necessarily their true opinion.

Much of the evaluation literature relating to IPE comprises 'black box' evaluations (Robson, 1993). In other words, we tend to know quite a bit about what is going into a project and are able to measure what is coming out, but are less sure about what actually happens in the middle and how these elements are related. Yet it is this middle bit – the workings inside the black box – that often determines what the outcomes of an intervention will be. We cannot presume that just because an intervention is designed in a particular way that it will run smoothly and that learners (who could potentially hold quite different values and principles) will react to it in the same way. Moreover, such an approach presumes that these programmes undergo little or no change during the period of study. Some researchers (Reeves, 2000) have favoured process-based research over before-and-after approaches in an attempt to examine all the factors that are going on within the process of an intervention. However, in practical terms this can end up being quite a time-consuming process, and if done solely on a qualitative basis lack the 'robust' evidence of effectiveness that is often sought within the fields of health and social care. For this reason some researchers have sought mixed method approaches that combine both quantitative and qualitative data and have gained a more nuanced view of the inputs, processes and outcomes (see, for example, Gilbert et al, 2000; Knapp et al, 2000; Reeves and Freeth, 2002). This has also led to slightly different questions being asked about IPE. Rather than asking just whether IPE 'works', a number of commentators (Hammick, 2000) have started to ask why it is effective, who it is effective for, when, and within what contexts.

Clearly these sorts of questions require very different approaches to the traditional gold standard (and often clinically influenced) RCTs and other controlled trials. These evaluation approaches are often known as 'method-led' approaches in that they presume that difficulties in evaluation result from methodological shortcomings, and that refinement of research methods alone will lead to the solutions (Chen, 1990). However, theory-led evaluation has become popular in recent years (for further discussion of theory-led and method-led evaluation, see Dickinson and O'Flynn, 2016). Rather than inferring causation from the input and outputs of a project, as experimentation does by excluding all other rival causal links, theory-led evaluation aims to map out the entire process (Pawson and Tilley, 1997). This allows the researcher to say with some confidence which parts of the programme worked and why, whether they would be applicable to different situations, and if there were any positive or negative effects that would otherwise not be anticipated (Birckmayer and Weiss, 2000). Theory-led evaluation has become particularly popular in relation to interventions that are complex and multifaceted (as IPE tends to be). One such theory-led approach is known as realistic evaluation (Pawson and Tilley, 1997), and this has been used to evaluate the IPE initiative illustrated in Box 3.4.

Realistic evaluation is characterised by the equation:

$$Context\ (C) + Mechanism\ (M) = Outcome\ (O)$$

This approach suggests that causal powers reside in mechanisms that are triggered when they are subject to specific contexts. When these causal powers are mobilised, they will produce certain outcomes. Contexts may be made up of any range of factors including history, geography, structures, culture, politics and so on, and they will change over time. Mechanisms refer not just to specific objects or individuals, but also to social relationships and specific actions. Mechanisms may therefore be observable, but they may also be hidden. Certain types of outcomes will only be produced when the context triggers the causal powers of mechanisms. Evaluators who employ such an approach therefore seek to uncover 'CMO configurations'. That is, they aim to uncover what kinds of contexts are needed to trigger specific mechanisms to produce a certain type of outcome (see Chapter 4 for an overview of the 'stepwise' approach to evaluation, which similarly aims to make firm statements about links between process factors and outcomes).

Box 3.4: Realistic evaluation and IPE evaluation

Steven et al (2007) employed a realistic evaluation approach to evaluate the Common Learning Programme in the North East. The research team used interview and observation methods among others in order to collect data on this programme that would allow them to look inside the 'black box'. The team suggest that in the quest for evidence-based policy and practice, particular forms of evidence and ways of knowing were elevated at the expense of overlooking others. Furthermore, they suggest that little attention was paid to the ways in which practice-based IPE actually took place, the processes involved and the role of context and its influence on outcomes. By adopting a realistic evaluation approach the team believed that these issues problems could be overcome.

Steven and colleagues outlined a number of contexts including different clinical settings and the range of participants involved. Mechanisms identified included the content of sessions and the procedures involved. Their findings indicated that discussions arose and evolved during IPE sessions in complex and unpredictable ways. Moreover, complex interplays arose between contexts, mechanisms and knowledge types. The team concluded that practice-based IPE was both complex and unpredictable, and for this reason, theory-led evaluation approaches such as realistic evaluation were more suited to these forms of settings.

Patsios and Carpenter (2010) examined the outputs and outcomes of inter-agency training to safeguard children in eight LSCBs in England. A review of documentation, observations of training sub-group meetings and a series of interviews with key stakeholders were used to assess how partner agencies carried out their statutory responsibilities to organise inter-agency training. Realistic evaluation was used to evaluate the mechanisms by which a central government mandate produced particular inter-agency training outputs (number of courses, training days) and joint working outcomes (effective partnerships). The authors concluded that government policy had played a key role in the mechanism and outputs of inter-agency training for joint working. It had fostered effective joint working through inter-agency training, which has the potential to create a better trained workforce to work together to safeguard children and to maintain their wellbeing. However, the generic guidelines offered in these policies have not resulted in homogeneous training organisation mechanisms across the various sites. Inter-agency training for joint working has triggered different organisational responses, producing different outcomes, which very much depended on the particular circumstances of the site. The effectiveness of the outputs and outcomes of inter-agency training was contingent on the context in which it was introduced. In short, what worked to produce effective organisation and delivery of inter-agency training in one site did not produce it uniformly across all others.

Carpenter et al (2007) suggest employing a 'stepwise' approach to the evaluation of process and outcomes. Although Carpenter and colleagues use this approach within a multidisciplinary postgraduate programme focused on the use of psychosocial intervention with mental health service users, we would argue that it is also suitable to use in IPE programmes more widely. Adopting a stepwise approach aims to avoid false inferences being made between specific practices and any effects that may have been observed. This multidimensional approach provides interrelated 'quality assurance' data on the structure, processes and outcomes of IPE, and enables evaluators to draw valid inferences about the effectiveness of a programme.

A stepwise approach involves at least one form of evidence at each step of the IPE programme. As Carpenter et al (2007, p 508) explain:

> This means that data are required about the trainees, which is correlated with training-related outcomes. It then necessitates some data on the training itself (eg adherence to programme specification in content and delivery), and then about the achievement of intended learning outcomes (eg knowledge about PSI [psychosocial intervention] techniques). These three logical steps in evaluation should lead on to a demonstration that any learning outcomes are transferred to the work environment, where any outcomes for service users and carers are obtained.

In other words, data is collected at each level of the Kirkpatrick-Barr et al (Kirkpatrick, 1967; Barr et al, 2000) outcome framework (outlined in Chapter 4) to ensure that any inferences that are made about outcomes directly follow on from the effects of the IPE programme and the influence of one level on the next, and are not due to any other possible extraneous forces.

Leaving aside the issue of methodologies that have been used to evaluate IPE initiatives for a moment, a key problem that researchers have encountered when attempting to draw out lessons from published evaluations is lack of information. This is partly a result of the academic process of reporting research findings. Journal articles are strictly limited in word length, and editors may ask for specific data to the exclusion of what might be quite crucial information. However, given the many different forms that IPE might take and the many things that may happen during the course of an IPE intervention, it is precisely this sort of documentary analysis that is essential in comparing programmes and uncovering generaliseable lessons. There have therefore been a number of calls imploring IPE evaluators to be more clear and transparent about the nature of the intervention, the context it took place in, who was involved, what educational models underpinned the intervention, how the data was analysed and so on (see, for example, Reeves, 2001). When writing up evaluations it is useful to bear this in mind and to try to include all such information, as it may be helpful to others in the future.

This issue of information actually overlaps with theory-led evaluation discussed previously. As Steven et al (2007) suggested, black box approaches often fail to outline a significant amount of information about the nature and the execution of IPE programmes. One approach that has been employed in order to help outline all the potential factors that might influence an IPE programme and any potential impacts that it might have is the '3P' model (originally illustrated by Freeth and Reeves, 2004). The 3Ps in this model are presage, process and product: where presage is the influence and constraint on the design and delivery of the programme; process is the delivery of the programme including interaction between learners and teachers, levels of engagement and so on; and the product is the outcomes of IPE (see Figure 3.1). This may be a useful model for evaluators of IPE to employ so they can classify the range of factors that may potentially have an impact on the programme and illustrate this to others who are unlikely to have the same in-depth knowledge of the particular context.

The model may also be helpful retrospectively in analysing why desired outcomes were not achieved. For example, Reeves and Freeth (2006) revisited data from an evaluation of a series of post-qualifying training workshops for community mental health teams. They wanted to understand why, in spite of an apparently successful event, none of the action plans developed by participants had been realised. The model helped them to appreciate a number of presage factors, specifically, time limitations, competing demands and funding restrictions.

Drawing on the various debates outlined here and the difficulties inherent in evaluating IPE projects, we end this chapter with a set of guidelines derived for IPE evaluation (see Box 3.5). It is worth re-iterating at this point that IPE evaluation is not easy – even for experienced researchers – and there is no 'right' way to do this and encapsulate all the complexity of such initiatives. Yet it is a crucial stage, not only in demonstrating the effectiveness of individual interventions and making these more effective and more appropriate to learners, but also in terms of providing an evidence base that can underpin IPE in a much more comprehensive fashion.

Figure 3.1: The 3P model of IPE

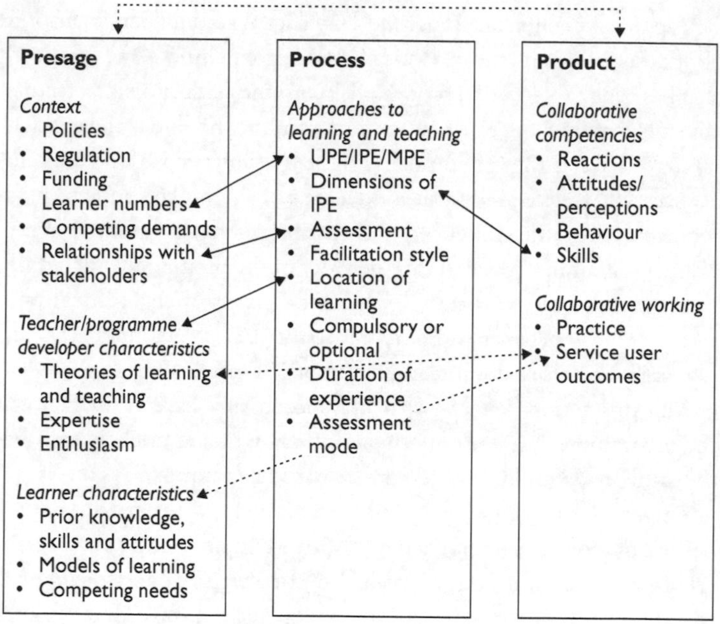

Presage	Process	Product
Context • Policies • Regulation • Funding • Learner numbers • Competing demands • Relationships with stakeholders *Teacher/programme developer characteristics* • Theories of learning and teaching • Expertise • Enthusiasm *Learner characteristics* • Prior knowledge, skills and attitudes • Models of learning • Competing needs	*Approaches to learning and teaching* • UPE/IPE/MPE • Dimensions of IPE • Assessment • Facilitation style • Location of learning • Compulsory or optional • Duration of experience • Assessment mode	*Collaborative competencies* • Reactions • Attitudes/ perceptions • Behaviour • Skills *Collaborative working* • Practice • Service user outcomes

Source: Adapted from Freeth and Reeves (2004)

Box 3.5: Guidelines for IPE evaluation

- If possible, plan the evaluation as part of the IPE planning process.
- Be clear about the aims of the intervention, the context it is taking place within, the resources you have available, and the boundaries of the intervention.
- Following on from the aims of the intervention, what is it you are trying to evaluate? What outcomes would you expect, and at what level? (Use the Kirkpatrick-Barr framework outlined in Chapter 4.) Are there any potential negatives or unanticipated impacts, and how would you detect them?
- Once you have determined the aims of the intervention and your evaluation, set yourself clear research questions.
- Use these specific questions to determine the methodology you will use for the evaluation. Is this the most appropriate approach you could use or would another model be more appropriate? Make sure you know why you have discounted other approaches.
- Use the methodology to guide who you involve within the evaluation, and include a theoretical basis for this sampling technique.
- Even if you cannot employ a controlled design, try to find a suitable comparison group of students, or service users, who do not experience the effects of the IPE programme. This applies to qualitative as well as quantitative evaluations: it is through comparisons that it is possible to tease out what makes a difference.
- If using outcome measures, use those that have previously been validated by other researchers (see Chapter 4 for a summary of these).
- Make sure that your qualitative or quantitative analytical approaches are consonant with the evaluation methodology you have used.
- When writing up, be clear who your audience is, what kinds of information they would need and the style of writing they would expect.
- When writing up, give a clear description of the intervention (the 3Ps), participation rates (including information on any withdrawals

and reasons for this), methodology employed, any limitations and potential future areas of research.

- Beyond any short-term impacts that may have been identified, what are the implications for longer-term outcomes? Will you continue to measure for future impact? Is there any scope to return and conduct a piece of work later?

Reflective exercises

1. Think of a range of ways in which service users might be involved in IPE programmes. What do you think the positives and negatives of these different approaches might be for (a) the service users themselves, (b) students, (c) facilitators of the programme and (d) overall impact of the programme? If you can, compare your thoughts with a colleague.

2. Think about an IPE programme you have been involved with or have read about. What practical steps would you take to involve service users in this programme? What do you think this would achieve?

3. Make a list of all the potential obstacles to sustaining and implementing learning from IPE programmes in practice. Which do you think could be most easily overcome? Which do you think would be most difficult to overcome? If you can, compare your thoughts with a colleague.

4. Read an account of an IPE programme (either in a journal or report). Does this contain all the information you need to understand the programme and evaluation? Is there any information missing that you think could be useful? Do you think the evaluation approach is appropriate to the subject? What would you do to improve this?

5. Think about a programme of IPE that you have either experienced as a learner or as a teacher/facilitator, or about a programme that you are planning. Preferably with a colleague, go through the guidelines in Box 3.5 and plan an evaluation from scratch. Assume, for the moment, that resources are no object to realising your plans!

Further reading and resources

- The European InterProfessional Education Network (EIPEN) in health and social care aims to share and develop effective interprofessional vocational training curricula, methods and materials for improving collaborative practice and multiagency working in health and social care. Readers may find this a useful site to obtain examples and key lessons when planning IPE programmes: www.eipen.org/
- The Centre for Interprofessional Practice is based at the University of East Anglia and facilitates the continuing professional development of health and social care teams. The centre works with pre- and post-registration health and social care professionals to make multidisciplinary environments more effective: www.uea.ac.uk/centre-for-interprofessional-practice
- Readers seeking further information on involving service users in educational programmes may find the Social Care Institute for Excellence's *Involving service users and carers in social work education* a useful and practical introduction (Levin, 2004).
- Readers seeking further information on types of evaluation and methods for evaluating IPE initiatives may find Dickinson and O'Flynn's book in this series instructive (2016). Also helpful are Freeth et al's *Effective interprofessional education* (2005a) and *Evaluating interprofessional education* (2005b).

4

Useful frameworks and concepts

While previous chapters have provided an overview of the aims of IPE and guidance for readers in terms of how to plan, run and evaluate IPE programmes, these have often also raised a number of key questions about the nature of IPE and to some extent problematised the issue. This final substantive chapter is slightly different and seeks to develop previous discussions in order to summarise a series of useful theoretical frameworks and approaches that students and educators may use to help unpick some of the themes and issues highlighted earlier.

Theories underpinning IPE

Reeves and Hean (2013) argued that an understanding and application of theory is necessary for appreciating the nature of interprofessional education, practice and care. They cited an influential review by Freeth and colleagues (2005a) to support their view that curriculum design for IPE and its evaluation had failed to employ theory in an explicit manner. As we suggested earlier, IPE programmes have generally suffered from a failure to be explicit about the nature of educational theories by which they are underpinned. Yet if IPE is to be considered a substantive and informed practice, it is important that its programmes are clearly and explicitly supported by educational theory. This section outlines some of the main educational theories that are associated with IPE, and the implications of such approaches in practice.

Adult learning theory

In Chapter 1 we outlined some of the main features of adult learning theory (Knowles, 1990) In order to produce an effective IPE initiative based on adult learning theory, there are several assumptions that need to be satisfied (see Box 4.1).

Box 4.1: Assumptions underlying adult learning theory

- Adult learners need to know the relevance of what they need to learn before undertaking to learn it.
- Adults prefer responsibility for their decisions and desire to be viewed as capable of self-direction.
- Adults accumulate a great volume of experience, which represents a rich resource for learning and necessitates individualisation of learning strategies.
- Adults become ready to learn things when they need to know them in order to cope effectively with real-life situations.
- Adults have a task-centred orientation to learning and like to feel free to focus on the task or problem.
- Students can work collaboratively and in dialogue with others with mutual trust and respect, both peers and lecturers, to shape, elaborate and deepen understanding.
- While adults are responsive to some external motivators, their most potent motivators are internal.

Source: Adapted from Craddock et al (2006, p 230)

IPE programmes that take account of these assumptions need to make sure that their desired outcomes are also those of the learners. Where there is a mismatch, learners may not be motivated to take part in the process. Programmes will also need to be learner-centred, experience-based, problem-orientated and collaborative in their approach, which clearly lends itself more to some modes of delivery and assessment than others. Barr et al (2005) summarise strategies used in IPE to facilitate adult learning. With a few notable exceptions such as PBL, these terms are not often employed in descriptions in the literature and they often overlap to a considerable extent. Nevertheless, it is useful to distinguish the following:

- *PBL, also known as EAL* (see, for example, Reeves and Freeth, 2002). Students work in small interprofessional groups examining service user-centred scenarios or case studies. These make use of triggers that stimulate student enquiry into relevant subject areas, typically allowing students to research information from their own disciplines that they share at subsequent group meetings. The idea is that students work cooperatively as an interprofessional team in order to achieve both subject-based learning outcomes and transferable teamwork skills. The pedagogy underpinning this approach has much in common with guided discovery learning (see, for example, O'Halloran et al, 2006). This emphasises self-directed learning supported by study guides where understanding is reinforced through its application in problem-oriented, task-based and work-related experiences.
- *Simulation-based learning* (see, for example, Wakefield et al, 2003), such as role-play with other students, actors or volunteer service users, is common within professional education. It may therefore be used in common foundation courses in communication and interviewing skills. Simulation provides a relatively safe context in which students can practice skills and receive feedback in a way that would not be possible with real service users. Simulation may be used in IPE in more elaborate role-play exercises in which participants take on their professional roles engaging in a simulated case conference or a court session (including lawyers).
- *Practice-based learning* (see, for example, Reeves et al, 2002) is where students take responsibility for working in a real-life setting on a clinical/placement as members of a team with supervision from mentors, for example, on a ward or in a community setting where they may also engage in a project designed to benefit the local population.

- *Exchange-based learning* (see, for example, Foy et al, 2002) emphasises the participants exchanging their views and experiences and learning from each other in so doing. Many programmes use this approach as a structured introductory exercise, inviting participants to share in pairs or small groups. But of course the whole programme may be seen as an opportunity to exchange. Hearing about the experiences of service users and carers (see, for example, Turner et al, 2000) may also be seen as exchange-based learning, although this should really be reserved for situations in which the students also share their experiences of caring.

- *Observation-based learning* (Guest et al, 2002) is a variant on exchange-based learning, where a member of a profession shadows a member of another profession to see what they do and how they do it. The aim here is to learn about the other professional's roles and responsibilities. In order to achieve this, there should be opportunities built in to question the person you are shadowing and to discuss your observations in uniprofessional or interprofessional groups (there is a case for both). Mutual learning will be enhanced if each person takes a turn to shadow the other.

- *Electronically enhanced learning (e-learning)* has seen recent growth in respect to IPE. Barr et al (2011) set out five overlapping uses: access to information through the internet; virtual learning environments and tools to enhance reflective learning such as e-portfolios; use of e-communication tools to enable synchronous discussion; electronic simulation and Web 2.0 technologies; and social networking.

- *Blended learning* combines e-learning, which can occur at different times to suit individual student needs (asynchronous) with face-to-face interactions between participants, which can use e-communication systems such as Skype. This approach has considerable practical advantages if timetabling and/or geographical distance make it difficult to meet. Carbonaro et al (2008) found that outcomes for blended learning students in achieving team process skills were no different to face-to-face students and a somewhat more positive achievement of course learning objectives.

Social psychology of IPE: using contact theory in programme planning

From a psychological perspective, the most striking feature of IPE is that it brings together two or more groups for a period of group interaction. Participants are there *because* of their membership of a professional group, or as students on their way to becoming members of a profession. The study of social identities and intergroup behaviour is very much the province of social psychology and, as Carpenter and Dickinson (2016) explain, the understanding and application of these theories can both increase the chances of IPE programmes having positive outcomes and reduce the chances of planned contact going badly wrong.

Wistow and Waddington (2006) vividly describe the differences in social and health models and underpinning values, suggesting that these can cause friction when professionals from different agencies are required to work together. Adult learning theory alone will be insufficient to address these issues, but an underlying assumption of many IPE initiatives is that if professions are brought together, they have the opportunity to learn about each other and dispel the negative stereotypes that are presumed to hamper interprofessional collaboration in practice. Much of the early work on the social psychology of intergroup contact was done by Allport (1954) and is known as 'contact theory'.

Allport accepted the 'common-sense' proposition that the best way to reduce hostility between groups was to bring them together, but he nevertheless argued that 'contact is not enough'. In other words, simply putting together a collection of students from different professions in the classroom – what we have defined in Chapter 1 as MPE – would not be enough to produce attitude change. Allport proposed as necessary conditions that the groups should have equal status within the contact situation, work on common goals, have the support of authorities (institutional support) and finally, that they should cooperate with each other. Allport's propositions have been tested in many real-life as well as experimental situations. A review of this literature by Hewstone and Brown (1986) identified four additional factors: first, that participants in the contact have positive expectations; second, that the joint work is successful; third, that there is a concern for similarities and differences between members of the groups; and finally, that the members of the conflicting groups who are brought together perceive each other as typical members of the other group and not just as exceptions to the stereotype. A limitation of the theory is that it does not specify *how* change will occur. While intergroup attitudes are influenced by many factors, including historical, social and political ones, cognitive processes, notably stereotyping, also play an important role.

Hewstone and Brown (1986) outlined the essential aspects of stereotyping. These are first, that other individuals are categorised, usually based on some observable characteristic such as gender, race or perhaps professional uniform. A set of attributes is then ascribed to most, if not all, of the members of that category. Everyone who belongs to that category is then assumed to be similar to each other and different from other groups. Thus outgroups (those groups of which we are not members) are generally seen as homogeneous while the ingroup (groups to which we perceive we belong) is seen as more diverse. Stereotypes generate expectations and we tend to 'see' behaviour that confirms our expectations even when it is absent. As Hewstone and Brown (1986) put it, contact situations can easily become self-fulfilling prophecies. This may explain why contact alone is not enough to change intergroup attitudes.

Pettigrew (1998) proposed that contact improves attitudes between groups by providing opportunities to learn about outgroups. Not surprisingly, Rothbart and John (1985) showed that positive change only occurred when the outgroup's behaviour was not in line with the traditional stereotype (for example, that the surgeons taking part in IPE revealed themselves to be caring and not at all arrogant), but also that these outgroup members were seen as being typical (of surgeons in general). Similarly, contact may provide insight into how others see us, and this may lead to a reappraisal of how we see ourselves. For example, we may not have thought about our own profession as being particularly knowledgeable, but faced by other professionals who clearly think this, we may revise our opinions. Furthermore, perceptions of one's own group, the 'ingroup', are reshaped in this way; this can lead to a less narrow-minded view of the outgroup ('they obviously value what I have to say. Maybe they are not as ignorant as I first thought').

The role of emotions in intergroup encounters and participants' anxiety should be recognised. For example, Carpenter and Hewstone (1996) reported that some medical students were apprehensive about IPE sessions with social work students, anticipating 'doctor bashing'; conversely, social work students acknowledged apprehension because they were 'prejudiced' about doctors. Similarly, Ajjawi et al (2009) documented dental students' discomfort and marginalisation in IPE with medical students. And it may be proposed that positive emotions can be facilitated by the development of friendships between participants.

Generalisation beyond the immediate contact situation is vital if the impact of intergroup contact is to have lasting consequences. Of course, when applied to IPE it is hoped that positive attitude change about other professionals engendered through the programme will extend to other professionals with whom they work. The question is, how to achieve generalisation?

Two models have been suggested, both forms of the contact hypothesis and based on social identity theory (Tajfel and Turner, 1986). Tajfel and Turner proposed that we derive our identity from our membership of social groups and further, that we prefer to have a positive rather than a negative identity. Therefore, it is argued that we will perceive the ingroup more positively than the outgroup. Social identity theory would emphasise a group-based rather than individualistic approach to achieving integration and collaboration between professionals in health and social care (Kreindler et al, 2012). For example, instead of nurses and social workers perceiving themselves by professional group, a common categorisation of 'mental health workers' could be emphasised during intergroup contact situations. However, this new identity is unlikely to be accepted unless it was more positively valued than the original professional identity. Thus the identity 'psychological therapist' might be more attractive than 'mental health worker' because it suggests higher status.

Hewstone and Brown (1986) alternatively proposed that salience is maintained for the original groups and contact conditions are optimised. This model attempts to maximise the group nature of the contact as opposed to the personal nature. In this way, contact should promote generalisation across members of the target outgroup. Hewstone and Brown argued that it is important to protect the distinctiveness of groups involved in contact for two reasons. First, the salience of group boundaries can promote generalisation across members of the outgroup and second, each group should be seen as distinct in terms of the expertise and experience it brings to the contact situation. This should result in 'mutual intergroup differentiation' in which groups recognise and value each other's strengths and weaknesses.

Hewstone and Brown went on to assert that a mutual recognition of superiorities and inferiorities would be reflected in intergroup stereotypes. They hypothesised that after intergroup contact that emphasised mutual intergroup differentiation, each group would view itself positively and hold positive stereotypes of outgroups. The positive stereotypes of the outgroup would be consistent with those groups' own views of their profession (autostereotypes). In summary, this model argues that after successful intergroup contact, each group is seen as it wishes to be seen, and desired differences between groups are highlighted.

The literature reviewed thus far suggests some conditions for changing attitudes in IPE that we perceive as an intergroup encounter. First, there should be institutional support for participation; this should be from the people or organisation that the participants feel to be influential. For pre-qualification students this may be college tutors; for practising professionals, it may be their colleagues, managers and/ or professional bodies. Second, participants should have positive expectations. While it is important that similarities between the groups are emphasised, differences should also be explored. The contact situation should emphasise the equality of participants on the programme even if they have a different status outside (for example, doctors and nurses). The learning atmosphere should be cooperative rather than competitive. Additionally, joint work should be successful if intergroup attitudes are to improve.

For positive attitude change to then be generalised from the outgroup members involved in the contact to all outgroup members, the members involved in the contact situation must be perceived as typical. Thus, for example, the nurses on a programme should be seen as representative of nurses whom social workers and occupational therapists encounter in their day-to-day working if they are to change their attitudes to nurses in general. The contact situation must also allow for both intergroup and interpersonal contact so that participants can relate to outgroup members both as individuals and as representatives of their professions.

Carpenter and Hewstone reported three empirical investigations of attitude change in IPE for social work, medical and nursing students at the University of Bristol (Hewstone et al, 1994; Carpenter, 1995a, 1995b; Carpenter and Hewstone, 1996). The programmes, which were compulsory, were designed in the light of the theoretical framework described above in that every effort was made to incorporate the 'contact variables' into their design. In these programmes, mutual intergroup differentiation was evident: participants were prepared to acknowledge the superiority to the outgroup on some dimensions. For example, Carpenter (1995b) reported that both medical and nursing students demonstrated strong positive and negative stereotypes: nurses were seen, by themselves and by the medics, as caring, dedicated and good communicators, whereas the medics were seen as confident by themselves and by the nurses. It is worth noting that these stereotypes were already strong despite neither group having at the time commenced their professional careers. This suggests that stereotypes are formed at a very early stage. Hind et al (2003) and Hean et al (2006), investigating health and social work undergraduates, and Mandy et al (2004), with physiotherapy and podiatry students, similarly found that clear and distinct professional stereotypes were present at an early stage of professional development.

At the end of the Bristol programmes, participants reported increased understanding of the knowledge and skills, roles and duties of the other profession. Further, there was encouraging evidence of changes in interprofessional stereotypes, with a reduction in the attribution of negative characteristics to the outgroups and an increase in those characteristics that were valued by the outgroup members. For example, social work students saw medical students as more caring and less detached, while the medics saw the social workers as less 'dithering' and gave them higher ratings for breadth of life experience. These positive results were associated with students' ratings of the design features of the programme, which supported the relevance of the contact hypothesis to IPE. Nevertheless, Carpenter and Hewstone point out that for one in five students attitudes actually worsened, which reminds us that individuals are different, and that what works for some does not for others.

These programmes were short (between one day and one week), involved students rather than qualified and experienced professionals, and the outcomes were not followed up into practice. In other words, changes in attitudes may have been insubstantial and transitory.

Carpenter and colleagues subsequently investigated stereotypes and stereotype change in a much longer (two-year, part-time) programme of IPE (described in Box 3.3). There was considerable evidence of professional stereotyping at the start of the programme, but in spite of the length of the programme, little evidence of change in these stereotypes at the end of the first year; positive stereotypes were not strengthened appreciably, nor were negative stereotypes reduced.

Having examined possible reasons for the absence of stereotype change, Barnes et al (2000b) concluded first, that the students tended not to see fellow course members as 'typical' and therefore did not generalise their positive experiences of fellow students to their professions as a whole. In particular, students considered that the main differences between themselves and their colleagues who did not elect to join the programme were their open mindedness and willingness to change.

Second, there was evidence that students did not perceive the programme to provide the conditions for positive attitude change required by contact theory. In particular, the requirements to explore differences as well as to emphasise similarities was not met, and there was little joint work involving participants from other professions. This was confirmed by participant observation of the teaching sessions. Another point to consider is that the programme was part-time, with students returning to their workplaces for the rest of the week; here, their pre-existing stereotypes might be reinforced.

Carpenter and Dickinson (2016) conclude from their review of the evidence: (1) that professional stereotypes, both positive and negative, are readily elicited from health and social work students and professionals, and also that there is a possibly a general consensus as to what these are; (2) there is some evidence that these stereotypes can be changed, at least in the short term, and with prequalification students; (3) these changes seem to be associated with the 'contact variables' (Hewstone and Brown, 1986), although we cannot say which of these conditions are 'essential' and which are 'facilitative'; and (4) in the relative absence of these conditions, attitude change *may* not take place or be generalised to the workplace. The perceived typicality of course participants seems to be quite important.

Carpenter and Dickinson (2016) argue that educators should use contact theory in IPE programme planning. In Box 4.2 their specific recommendations are presented. There is as much to learn from unsuccessful examples of programmes as the successful ones, so we have referenced these.

Box 4.2: Using contact theory in IPE programme design

- Try to ensure that participants in the programme have *equal status* and are not marginalised (Carpenter and Hewstone, 1996; Ajjawi et al, 2009). Remember that status derives from the expertise and experience as well as the length and prestige of qualifying courses.
- Design small group classroom exercises (Barnes et al, 2000b; Mohaupt et al, 2012) or tasks to be undertaken on practice placements or 'training wards' (Reeves and Freeth, 2002) in which participants see *common goals*, agree on their importance and engage in joint work.
- Ensure that *institutional support* for the programme is apparent to the participants (Carpenter, 1995b; Furness et al, 2012). Indicators are the involvement of high status staff, good quality teaching facilities and prominent place in the curriculum, as well as formal assessment of learning.
- Engender *positive expectations* of the programme. Talk to student representatives, recruit 'ambassadors' who have previously experienced the programme and prepare good promotional material (Furness et al, 2012).
- Encourage *generalisation* by asking participants to assume their professional discipline in IPE workshops (Barnes et al, 2000b). Note that this can be difficult for inexperienced students who may not know enough to do this convincingly.
- Ensure that participants explore differences as well as similarities in professional roles, knowledge, skills and values (Barnes et al, 2000b).
- Balance the numbers of participants as far as possible. A solo representative of a profession may feel outnumbered and oppressed by the majority, particularly if this person also feels disadvantaged by gender and ethnicity (Ajjawi et al, 2009).

Whether or not the objectives of an IPE programme are explicitly to tackle interprofessional stereotyping and promote attitude change, it is crucial to recognise and plan how to deal with the intergroup aspects of the encounter. Barr et al (2005, p 124) argue that when developing IPE initiatives it is crucial to choose between these models in distinguishing what the programme is trying to achieve in terms of changing professional identities. Although within the partnership literature different professional identities and values are often represented as being a barrier to more effective working, they can also hold considerable value. Much early partnership literature talked about the value of blurring roles so that generic workers might take on tasks regardless of professional boundaries (and this is reflected in policy, as seen earlier), but some commentators have indicated that this might, in fact, be detrimental to both organisational and individual performance (see, for example, Rushmer and Pallis, 2002; Rushmer, 2005). There is more discussion of roles and blurring of boundaries in the teamworking text in this series (see Jelphs et al, 2016).

As suggested earlier, this brief overview of theories is by no means an exhaustive list, and many other different approaches to educational theory exist within the literature. However, it is crucial that coherent IPE programmes are underpinned by an appropriate educational theory, and that this is consonant with the aims, forms and method of that initiative. Without this congruence the IPE intervention may not be as effective as predicted – both in terms of impacts on learners, but also in terms of outcomes for service users.

Outcomes of IPE

Kirkpatrick (1967) originally set out a model of learning outcomes. The model outlines four stages in terms of changing practice: behaviour, learning, reaction and results. Essentially what Kirkpatrick argues is that learners who are satisfied and react positively to the learning experience are more likely to be motivated to learn. This does not necessarily mean they will definitely do so, but a negative reaction is not likely to motivate individuals to learn. Successful learning will change attitudes and improve knowledge and, if this changes behaviour in the workplace, may improve practice. However, Kirkpatrick also notes a series of guiding principles that underpin this model, namely, that:

- outcomes in each of the areas are not hierarchical;
- the aim is to encourage more holistic and comprehensive evaluations to better inform future policy and development;
- there is acknowledgement that at each level it becomes progressively more difficult to gather trustworthy data on the educational intervention.

A modified version of Kirkpatrick's model – the Kirkpatrick-Barr framework of outcomes (see Table 4.1) – has been quite widely used within the IPE literature (see, for example, Barr et al, 2000; Freeth et al, 2002; Carpenter et al, 2006). Given the comments in the previous chapters regarding the many different impacts that IPE may produce and the importance of rigorous evaluation for the IPE movement, this framework is useful in that it provides a consistent classification of outcomes. It identifies outcomes at four separate levels (two of which have two separate impacts). Depending on what it is that IPE programmes have been set up to achieve, they may test for outcomes

Table 4.1: Kirkpatrick-Barr et al's (2000) framework of outcomes

1. Reaction	Learners' views on the learning experience and its interprofessional nature
2a. Modification of attitudes/perceptions	Changes in reciprocal attitudes or perceptions between participant groups. Changes in perception or attitude towards the value and/or use of team approaches to caring for specific client group
2b. Acquisition of knowledge/skills	Including knowledge and skills linked to interprofessional collaboration
3. Behavioural change	Identifies individuals' transfer of interprofessional learning to their practice setting and changed professional practice
4a. Change in organisational practice	Wider changes in the organisation and delivery of care
4b. Benefits to service users	Improvements in health or wellbeing of service users

Source: Barr et al (2000)

at some or all of these levels in order to demonstrate impact. Box 4.3 gives examples illustrating where this framework has been used to evaluate the outcomes of IPE and the types of measures used to detect these outcomes.

Box 4.3: Examples of levels of outcomes and measures

An evaluation to uncover level 1 outcomes would simply test whether learners enjoyed the experience, and this tends to be measured by a questionnaire rating learner satisfaction or enjoyment (examples of studies that have sought to examine changes in outcomes at this level include Doyle et al, 2003; Ker et al, 2003).

Studies to examine whether level 2a outcomes have been affected would be seeking to examine whether attitudes and perceptions have changed towards other professional groups or in relation to working in teams with other professionals. Again, this could be done by a questionnaire, and there are some available that are validated for these situations (see, for example, Carpenter, 1995a; Barnes et al, 2000a; Lindqvist et al, 2005; Lidskog et al, 2007).

Analysing changes in level 2b outcomes involves determining whether the collaborative skills or knowledge of learners has changed and again, this is often done via a questionnaire. Such questionnaires aim to determine whether individuals understand the roles and responsibilities of other professionals any better, whether they have developed teamwork skills and whether they have improved their knowledge of the nature of teamwork (see, for example, Farrell et al, 2001; Kwan et al, 2006).

Level 3 outcomes relate to behavioural change, and there is a range of different ways to examine alterations in these outcomes. Clearly, again, questionnaires may be employed, but there is a risk that learners indicate changes because they feel there should be some change when, in fact, little has changed. One possibility is to seek validation from the learner's line manager (see, for example, Barnes et al, 2006). Observational approaches or diary-based analysis approaches might also be used to see how often professionals communicate or cooperate with other professionals (see, for example, Morey et al, 2002).

Looking for changes in level 4a outcomes involves detecting alterations in organisational practice. This may again be done by a questionnaire, but has also been tracked by changes in referral practices, searching patient records, cost-effectiveness analysis, working practices and so on (see, for example, Baker et al, 1995; Bailey, 2002).

Level 4a and b changes involve impacts on the lives of service users. There are various means by which this may be detected including clinical or functional outcomes, service user satisfaction, days of institutional care used, service user life skills, emergency hospital readmissions and length of stay (see, for example, Treadwell et al, 2002; Carpenter et al, 2006; Strasser, 2008).

Thannhauser et al (2010) reviewed 23 self-report measures of IPE and collaboration that are listed in their paper. They present published evidence of the reliability and validity of the scales, information about the samples used in their development and a description of the type of scale, number of items and the factors each are intended to measure. These are aimed at detecting modification of attitudes and perceptions (level 2a), and reflect the development of IPE described in Chapter 2 and, especially, the predominant focus of university-based pre-qualifying IPE on interprofessional attitudes. They comment that psychometric information is often quite limited, and that some measures have only been used by the developers, so we do not know how they work in different contexts. Thannhauser and her colleagues focus on two quite widely used measures, the Readiness for Interprofessional Learning Scale (RIPLS) (Parsell and Bligh, 1998) and the related Interdisciplinary Education Perception Scale (IEPS) (Luecht et al, 1990). While the first measures attitudes to IPE itself, the second focuses on interprofessional collaboration, specifically 'competency and autonomy', 'perceived need for cooperation', and perception of actual cooperation'. Since their publication, McFadyen and his colleagues (McFadyen et al, 2006, 2007) have revised both scales, and they have been used in a longitudinal study of pre-registration students on an IPE programme in Scotland (McFadyen et al, 2010).

A similar set of self-report scales has been developed by Pollard et al (2004, 2005), referred to as the UWE Interprofessional Questionnaire. The scales are designed to measure attitudes to interprofessional learning, interprofessional interaction and communication and teamwork. They were used in the UWE outcomes study, summarised earlier, in Box 2.7.

Self-report measures are generally considered suitable for measuring attitudes and perceptions, but inadequate for measuring skills (level 2b). Thus Flaherty et al (2003) used five case scenarios in the measurement of teamwork skills. Student teams were tasked with developing an interprofessional care plan and trained raters scored their responses. There do not appear to be any instruments that claim to measure the transfer of interprofessional learning to the workplace (level 3). Asking participants to report on the extent to which they implemented their learning is of limited value if we do not have a pre-course measure. Also, it is difficult to define 'behaving interprofessionally' as precisely as, for example, using a new therapy.

Specialist post-qualifying programmes, particularly those focused on service-based team training, may consider using measures of team functioning to assess organisational changes (level 4a); examples, however, are few (see, for example, Healey et al, 2006; Oliver et al, 2007).

Some post-qualifying programmes concerned to assess benefits for service users (level 4b) have measured improvements in the quality of care in terms of subjective 'user satisfaction', and in some cases, objective counts of 'adverse events', such as clinical errors (Morey et al, 2002) and infections (Horbar et al, 2001). Whether service users would see the reduction in these as the *primary* outcome of care is a moot point. 'User satisfaction' can be a bland indicator that does not tell us very much, but questionnaires that ask about specific aspects of care and that are developed with service user input are likely to be much more sensitive to change and group comparison. Thus, for the University of Birmingham mental health study (as described earlier in Box 3.3), Barnes et al (2000a) worked with mental health service users to develop a questionnaire specifically to assess the 'user-defined outcomes' of IPE. This was then used to compare the quality of care provided by students who had been on the programme with those in another area who had not (Barnes et al, 2006).

However, most people would consider the most robust evidence of benefits to service users is of objective improvements in their health conditions, social functioning and quality of life. These can be measured for a whole range of service users using standardised measures. This was done in the Birmingham study of IPE for mental health (Carpenter et al, 2006) and in its replication elsewhere (Carpenter et al, 2007), where the researchers found greater improvement in the service users whose case workers had received training than those in the comparison group. However, in this case we must be careful about attributing measurable outcomes to IPE: we cannot claim that it was IPE that made the difference – similar positive outcomes for this group have been seen in psychosocial intervention programmes that do not stress IPE (Leff et al, 2001). The only way to attribute measured benefits unequivocally to IPE would be to make a direct comparison with UPE in an RCT with both trainees and service users randomised – not an easy task, as we have tried to demonstrate throughout this text!

Reflective exercises

1. Think about the assumptions underlying adult learning (see Box 4.1). Reflect on them in the light of your own experiences of learning. Do they hold true for you?

2. What implications do these factors hold for the design of an IPE programme? What things would you try to incorporate as a result of these factors? What things would you try not to do?

3. Think of an IPE programme you have experience of or have read about. What level of outcomes was this programme intended to produce? Did you think it achieved these? Were any data collected in order to evaluate these outcomes?

4. Use the questions in Box 4.2 to examine the extent to which the contact variables were present in this programme. What could have been done to improve the intergroup interaction?

5. Look back to the plans you made for evaluating a programme of IPE from the reflective exercises at the end of Chapter 3. Using the Kirkpatrick-Barr et al framework (see Table 4.1), review the outcomes you would seek to measure. Having defined your outcomes, consider the outcome measures mentioned and which would be most appropriate to use. Obtain the papers cited and review the content of the measures. Do you think the questions or statements measure what they are supposed to? Do you think they would be acceptable to the participants on the programme?

Further reading and resources

This chapter has indicated a wide range of key texts and resources that are summarised in the relevant sections. We would suggest that readers explore those that are relevant to their specific interests in conjunction with others identified throughout the book.

5

Recommendations for policy and practice

Drawing on the questions, summaries and frameworks set out in this book, there are a series of practical recommendations and potential warnings that arise, for both policy and practice.

For policy-makers

- Governments need to be clearer about what they expect IPE to deliver. IPE can, and should, play a major role in preparing professionals to work collaboratively to the ultimate benefit of service users and carers. But it is no substitute for removing the structural barriers to partnership working and providing local organisations with clear guidance about how they might go about working in partnerships.
- As a practical step, it would be helpful for policy-makers to adopt clear definitions of the various forms of learning involving more than one professional group, including the CAIPE definition of IPE.
- It is important to be clear about the motivation for, and goals of, IPE initiatives. Professionals and students accept the need to know about each other, and about how they can work together more effectively. Professional identities are important, and professionals may be more cautious if they perceive the goal as being role substitution. The notion of flexibility in career pathways may not be received with enthusiasm.
- IPE cannot simply be treated as an add-on to existing programmes of education and training. Neither can it be simply restricted to either pre- or post-qualification students. If health and social care organisations are to work together more effectively in practice, then

IPE needs to play an integral role in the education of professionals today and in the future. IPE should therefore be mandatory for all professional courses in all HEIs.

- IPE needs to be evaluated effectively and evidence of best practice needs to be shared between health and social care organisations. However, evaluation needs to go beyond whether IPE 'works' or not. Given that different types of IPE are driven by different aims and goals, we need to ask what forms of IPE work for which kinds of professionals, when and how. We need research that compares the outcomes of UPE and IPE so that we can know the circumstances in which IPE is an appropriate learning approach and when others may be more effective.

- We do not yet have any evidence that pre-qualifying learning of common 'foundation skills', such as communication skills, in interprofessional groups is effective. The evidence so far supports an emphasis on learning together about the process of working together in areas of common concern; this is the core focus of IPE.

- We recommend that, as in the case of social work education, governments stipulate that service users and carers must be involved in the development of IPE in HEIs, and in post-qualifying inter-agency training.

For education commissioners and managers in HEIs

- Elements of IPE should be built in to all professional courses and participation required by all students. Formal assessment of the interprofessional aspects of learning should be included for both university-based courses and clinical/practice placements.

- There is much that we still need to know about effective IPE, including when and how it should be delivered. Outcomes may be quite variable. Consequently, it is essential that programmes are carefully monitored and reviewed. We also recommend that, when commissioning programmes, money be set aside for formal evaluation, ideally by an external, independent evaluation team.

- Be clear that service users and carers should be involved in the planning and delivery of IPE, and ensure that money is available to pay for this at the proper rate.

For education managers, in addition

- It is important to recognise that developing and managing programmes of IPE is challenging and very time-consuming. It is essential to support programme directors with sufficient time and resources, including funding and administrative support. Encourage and enable staff to participate in national and international networks for IPE.
- Ensure that staff are recognised and rewarded for their contribution by senior managers as well as colleagues.
- Expect programme specifications and learning methods to be backed up by reference to underpinning theory.

For programme directors and staff involved in planning IPE

We very much hope that you have found the reflective exercises useful in stimulating your thinking about IPE. As a reminder, do not forget to:

- Engage and involve all the 'key players' and marshal your support (do not try and do it all by yourself!).
- Be explicit about the aims and objectives of your programme.
- Select and use underpinning adult learning theories to provide a firm foundation for your methods of learning and teaching.
- Ignore the psychology of intergroup behaviour at your peril! Instead, examine the contact variables and consider how you can maximise them in your programme.
- Prepare and support all those involved in teaching and facilitating, particularly service users and carers.
- Insist on proper arrangements for monitoring, review and formal evaluation.

For programme staff and facilitators, including service users and carers

- Ensure that you understand the principles behind the educational methods being planned and used on the programme, and that you are quite clear about its intended learning outcomes.
- Appreciate that IPE is generally more challenging to facilitate than UPE – but consequently, it can be even more rewarding.

For evaluators

- Remember that we need to know: what forms of IPE work for which kinds of professionals, when and how. Resist the simple request, 'does it work?'
- When planning your evaluation, make sure you open the 'black box': we need to know about context, processes and outcomes. Choose and use a conceptual model that makes sense to you.
- Plan and describe your evaluation methodology in terms of the Kirkpatrick-Barr et al framework of learning outcomes. Think about using the 'stepwise' approach and linking the different levels.
- Report negative as well as positive findings: in both cases, seek to understand context and mechanisms, otherwise the 2Ps (presage and process) that led to this 'product' are absent.

For students, both pre- and post-qualifying

- As with any learning opportunity, what you get out of it depends to a large extent on what you put in. So, express your views and share your experiences.
- Remember it is an exchange, so do not forget to listen and question as well.
- Expect to be challenged, but do not take challenges as a personal attack! Remember that other participants are likely to see you as representing your profession. See it as an opportunity (gently) to amend their negative stereotypes and to enhance positive ones.

- If the programme is not delivering – you are not learning, participants are not cooperating and becoming more not less antagonistic, the practice arrangements are breaking down and the online programme is not working – do not suffer in silence or vote with your feet. Let the staff and/or programme director know; that way the programme can be changed.
- And do not forget to complete those evaluation questionnaires and/ or attend that focus group or interview – the evaluator needs your data!

References

Ajjawi, R., Hyde, S., Roberts, C. and Nisbit, G. (2009) 'Marginalisation of dental students in a shared medical and dental education programme', *Medical Education*, vol 43, pp 238-45.

Allport, G.W. (1954) *The nature of prejudice*, Reading, MA: Addison-Wesley.

Anderson, E., Manek, N. and Davidson, A. (2006) 'Evaluation of a model for maximising interprofessional education in an acute hospital', *Journal of Interprofessional Care*, vol 20, pp 182-94.

Bailey, D. (2002) 'Training together – part II: an exploration of the evaluation of a shared learning programme on dual diagnosis for specialist drugs workers and approved social workers', *Social Work Education*, vol 21, pp 685-99.

Bailey, D. (2005) 'Using an action research approach to involving service users in the assessment of professional competence', *European Journal of Social Work*, vol 8, pp 165-79.

Baker, R., Sorrie, R., Reddish, S. and Hearnshaw, H. (1995) 'The facilitation of multi-professional clinical audit in primary health care teams – from audit to quality assurance', *Journal of Interprofessional Care*, vol 9, pp 237-44.

Baldwin, D.C. (1996) 'Some historical notes on interdisciplinary and interprofessional education and practice in health care in the USA', *Journal of Interprofessional Care*, vol 10, pp 173-87.

Balloch, S. and Taylor, M. (eds) (2001) *Partnership working: Policy and practice*, Bristol: Policy Press.

Barnes, D., Carpenter, J. and Bailey, D. (2000a) 'Partnerships with service users in interprofessional education for community mental health: a case study', *Journal of Interprofessional Care*, vol 14, pp 189-200.

Barnes, D., Carpenter, J. and Dickinson, C. (2000b) 'Interprofessional education for community mental health: attitudes to community care and professional stereotypes', *Journal of Interprofessional Care*, vol 19, pp 565-83.

Barnes, D., Carpenter, J. and Dickinson, C. (2006) 'The outcomes of partnerships with mental health service users in interprofessional education: a case study', *Health and Social Care in the Community*, vol 14, pp 426-35.

Barr, H. (1994) *Perspectives on shared learning*, London: Centre for the Advancement of Interprofessional Education.

Barr, H. (1996) 'Ends and means in interprofessional education: towards a typology', *Education for Health*, vol 9, pp 341-52.

Barr, H. (1998) 'Competent to collaborate: towards a competency-based model for interprofessional education', *Journal of Interprofessional Care*, vol 12, pp 181-7.

Barr, H. (2000) 'Working together to learn together: learning together to work together', *Journal of Interprofessional Care*, vol 14, pp 177-9.

Barr, H. (2002) *Interprofessional education today, yesterday and tomorrow: A review*, London: Learning and Teaching Support Network, Centre for Health Sciences and Practice.

Barr, H. (2015) *Interprofessional education: The genesis of a global movement*, Fareham: Centre for the Advancement of Interprofessional Education.

Barr, H. and Low, H. (2012) *Interprofessional learning in pre-registration education courses: A CAIPE guide for commissioners and regulators of education*, London: CAIPE.

Barr, H. and Ross, F. (2006) 'Mainstreaming interprofessional education in the United Kingdom: a position paper', *Journal of Interprofessional Care*, vol 20, pp 96-104.

Barr, H., Helme, M. and D'Avray, L. (2011) *Developing interprofessional education in health and social care courses in the United Kingdom*, London: Higher Education Academy.

Barr, H., Helme, M. and D'Avray, L. (2014) *Review of interprofessional education in the United Kingdom, 1997-2013*, Fareham: Centre for the Advancement of Interprofessional Education.

Barr, H., Hammick, M., Koppel, I. and Reeves, S. (1999) 'Evaluating interprofessional education: two systematic reviews for health and social care', *British Educational Research Journal*, vol 25, pp 533-44.

Barr, H., Hammick, M., Freeth, D., Koppel, I. and Reeves, S. (2000) *Evaluating interprofessional education: A UK review for health and social care*, London: British Education Research Association/ Centre for the Advancement of Interprofessional Education.

Barr, H., Koppel, I., Reeves, S., Hammick, M. and Freeth, D. (2005) *Effective interprofessional education: Argument, assumption and evidence*, Oxford: Blackwell Publishing.

Barrett, G., Greenwood, R. and Ross, K. (2003) 'Integrating interprofessional education into 10 health and social care programmes', *Journal of Interprofessional Care*, vol 17, pp 293-301.

Barrett, G., Sellman, D. and Thomas, J. (eds) (2005) *Interprofessional working in health and social care: Professional perspectives*, Basingstoke: Palgrave.

Benson, D. and Jordan, A. (2011) 'What have we learned from policy transfer research? Dolowitz and Marsh revisited', *Political Studies Review*, vol 9, no 3, pp 366-78.

Birckmayer, J.D. and Weiss, C.H. (2000) 'Theory-based evaluation in practice. What do we learn?', *Evaluation Review*, vol 24, pp 407-31.

Brandt, B., May, N.L., King, J.A. and Chioreso, C. (2014) 'A scoping review of interprofessional collaborative practice and education using the lens of the triple aim', *Journal of Interprofessional Care*, vol 28, no 5, pp 393-9.

CAIPE (Centre for the Advancement of Interprofessional Education) (1996) *Principles of interprofessional education*, London: CAIPE.

Campbell, J. and Johnson, C. (1999) 'Trend spotting: fashions in medical education', *British Medical Journal*, vol 318, p 1275.

Carbonaro, M., King, S., Taylor, E. et al (2008) 'Integration of e-learning technologies in an interprofessional health science course', *Medical Teacher*, vol 30, pp 25-33.

Carpenter, J. (1995a) 'Doctors and nurses stereotype change in interprofessional education', *Journal of Interprofessional Care*, vol 9, pp 151-61.

Carpenter, J. (1995b) 'Interprofessional education for medical and nursing students: evaluation of a programme', *Medical Education*, vol 29, pp 265-75.

Carpenter, J. and Dickinson, C. (2016) 'Understanding interprofessional education as an intergroup encounter: The use of contact theory in programme planning', *Journal of Interprofessional Care*, vol 30, no 1, pp 103-8.

Carpenter, J. and Hewstone, M. (1996) 'Shared learning for doctors and social workers: evaluation of a programme', *British Journal of Social Work*, vol 26, pp 239-57.

Carpenter, J., Barnes, D. and Dickinson, C. (2006) 'Outcomes of interprofessional education for Community Mental Health Services in England: the longitudinal evaluation of a postgraduate programme', *Journal of Interprofessional Care*, vol 20, pp 145-61.

Carpenter, J., Milne, D., Lombardo, C. and Dickinson, C. (2007) 'Process and outcomes of training in psychosocial interventions in mental health: a stepwise approach to evaluation', *Journal of Mental Health*, vol 16, pp 505-20.

Chen, H.-T. (1990) *Theory-driven evaluations*, London: Sage Publications.

CIHC (Canadian Interprofessional Health Collaborative) and CPIS (Consortium pancanadien pour l'interprofessionnalisme en santé) (2010) *A national interprofessional competency framework* (www.cihc.ca/files/CIHC_IPCompetencies_Feb1210.pdf).

Clark, P.G. (1997) 'Values in health care professional socialisation: implications for geriatric education in interdisciplinary teamwork', *Gerontologist*, vol 37, pp 441-51.

Cooper, H. and Spencer-Dawe, E. (2006) 'Involving service users in interprofessional education narrowing the gap between theory and practice', *Journal of Interprofessional Care*, vol 20, pp 603-17.

Craddock, D., Borthwick, A. and McPherson, K. (2006) 'Interprofessional education in health and social care: fashion or informed practice?', *Learning in Health and Social Care*, vol 5, pp 220-42.

D'Amour, D. and Oandasan, I. (2005) 'Interprofessionality as the field of interprofessional practice and interprofessional education: An emerging concept', *Journal of Interprofessional Care*, Supplement 1, pp 8-20.

Daykin, N., Rimmer, J., Turton, P., Evans, S., Sanidas, M., Tritter, J. and Langton, H. (2002) 'Enhancing user involvement through interprofessional education in healthcare: the case of cancer services', *Learning in Health and Social Care*, vol 1, pp 122-31.

DH (Department of Health) (1998) *Partnership in action: New opportunities for joint working between health and social services*, London: DH.

DH (1999) *Making a difference: Strengthening the nursing, midwifery and health visiting contribution to health and healthcare*, London: DH.

DH (2000a) *The NHS Plan: A plan for investment, a plan for reform*, London: The Stationery Office.

DH (2000b) *Meeting the challenge: A strategy for allied health professionals*, London: DH.

DH (2001a) *Investment and reform for NHS staff – taking forward the NHS Plan*, London: DH.

DH (2001b) *A health service of all the talents: Developing the NHS workforce*, London: DH.

DH (2001c) *Learning from Bristol: The report of the public inquiry into children's heart surgery at Bristol Royal Infirmary, 1984-1995*, London: The Stationery Office.

DH (2002a) *Liberating the talents: Helping primary care trusts and nurses to deliver the NHS Plan*, London: DH.

DH (2002b) *Reform of social work education and training*, London: DH.

DH (2002c) *Primary care workforce planning framework*, London: DH.

DH (2006) *Reward and recognition: The principles and practice of service user payment and reimbursement in health and social care*, London: The Stationery Office.

DH (2013) *Integrated care: Our shared commitment*, London: DH.

Dickinson, H. and Carey, G. (2016) *Managing and leading in inter-agency settings* (2nd edn), Better Partnership Working series, Bristol: Policy Press.

Dickinson, H. and O'Flynn, J. (2016) *Evaluating outcomes in health and social care* (2nd edn), Better Partnership Working series, Bristol: Policy Press.

Dolowitz, D. and Marsh, D. (2000) 'Learning from abroad: The role of policy transfer in contemporary policy-making', *Governance*, vol 13, no 1, pp 5-24.

Doyle, M., Earnshaw, P. and Galloway, A. (2003) 'Developing, delivering and evaluating interprofessional clinical risk training in mental health services', *Psychiatric Bulletin*, vol 27, pp 73-6.

Dunston, R. (2015) *The 'inter-professional' in Australian health professional education: Current activity and recommendations for action*, Sydney, NSW: University of Technology.

Farrell, M., Ryan, S. and Langrick, B. (2001) 'Breaking bad news within a paediatric setting: an evaluation report of a collaborative education workshop to support health professionals', *Journal of Advanced Nursing*, vol 36, pp 765-75.

Finch, J. (2000) 'Interprofessional education and teamworking: a view from the education providers', *British Medical Journal*, vol 321, pp 1138-40.

Fineberg, I., Wenger, N. and Farrow, L. (2004) 'Interdisciplinary education: evaluation of a palliative care training intervention for pre-professionals', *Academic Medicine*, vol 79, pp 769-76.

Flaherty, E., Heyer, K. and Kane, R. (2003) 'Using case studies to evaluate students' ability to develop a geriatric interdisciplinary care plan', *Gerontology and Geriatrics Education*, vol 24, pp 63-74.

Fox, N. (1994) 'Self-directed approaches to multidisciplinary health studies', *Journal of Interprofessional Care*, vol 8, pp 247-54.

Foy, R., Tidy, N. and Hollis, S. (2002) 'Interprofessional learning in primary care: lessons from an action-learning programme', *British Journal of Clinical Governance*, vol 7, pp 40-4.

Freeth, D. and Reeves, S. (2004) 'Learning to work together: using the presage, process, product (3P) model to highlight decisions and possibilities', *Journal of Interprofessional Care*, vol 18, pp 43-56.

Freeth, D., Hammick, M., Koppel, I., Reeves, S. and Barr, H. (2002) *A critical review of evaluations of interprofessional education*, London: Learning and Teaching Support Network, Centre for Health Sciences and Practice.

Freeth, D., Hammick, M., Reeves, S., Koppel, I. and Barr, H. (2005a) *Effective interprofessional education: Development, delivery and evaluation*, Oxford: Blackwell Publishing.

Freeth, D., Reeves, S., Koppel, I., Hammick, M. and Barr, H. (2005b) *Evaluating interprofessional education: A self-help guide*, London: Higher Education Academy Health Sciences and Practice Network.

Fulbright-Anderson, K., Kubisch, A.C. and Connell, J.P. (1998) *New approaches to evaluating community initiatives: Theory, measurement and analysis*, Washington, DC: Aspen Institute.

Furness, P.J., Armitage, H.R. and Pitt, R. (2012) 'Qualitative evaluation of interprofessional learning initiatives in practice: application of the contact hypothesis', *International Journal of Medical Education*, vol 3, pp 83-91.

Gilbert, J., Camp, R., Cole, C., Bruce, C., Fielding, D. and Stanton, S. (2000) 'Preparing students for interprofessional teamwork in health care', *Journal of Interprofessional Care*, vol 14, pp 223-5.

Glasby, J. and Dickinson, H. (2014a) *A-Z of interagency working*, Basingstoke: Palgrave Macmillan.

Glasby, J. and Dickinson, H. (2014b) *Partnership working in health and social care* (2nd edn), Better partnership working series, Bristol: Policy Press.

Glendinning, C., Powell, M. and Rummery, K. (eds) (2002) *Partnerships, New Labour and the governance of welfare*, Bristol: Policy Press.

GMC (General Medical Council) (2009) *Tomorrow's doctors*, London: GMC.

Graham, J. and Wealthall, S. (1999) 'Interdisciplinary education for health professions: taking the risk forcommunity gain', *Focus on Health Professional Education: a Multi-disciplinary Journal*, vol 1, no 1, pp 49-69.

Guest, C., Smith, L., Bradshaw, M. and Hardcastle, W. (2002) 'Facilitating interprofessional learning for medical and nursing students in clinical practice', *Learning in Health and Social Care*, vol 1, pp 132-8.

Hammick, M. (1998) 'Interprofessional education: concept, theory and application', *Journal of Interprofessional Care*, vol 12, pp 323-32.

Hammick, M. (2000) 'Interprofessional education: evidence from the past to guide the future', *Medical Teacher*, vol 22, pp 461-7.

HCPC (Health and Care Professions Council) (2014) *Standards of education and training*, London: HCPC.

Healey, A., Undre, S. and Sevdalis, N. (2006) 'The complexity of measuring interprofessional teamwork in the operating theatre', *Journal of Interprofessional Care*, vol 20, pp 485-95.

Hean, S., Clark, J., Macleod, J., Adams, K. and Humphris, D. (2006) 'Will opposites attract? Similarities and differences in students' perceptions of the stereotype pro les of other health and social care professional groups', *Journal of Interprofessional Care*, vol 20, pp 162-81.

Herbert, C.P. (2005) 'Editorial', *Journal of Interprofessional Care*, vol 19, Supplement 1, pp 1-4.

Hewstone, M. and Brown, R. (1986) 'Contact is not enough; an intergroup perspective on the "contact hypothesis"', in M. Hewstone and R. Brown (eds) *Contact and conflict in intergroup encounters*, Oxford: Blackwell.

Hewstone, M., Carpenter, J., Franklyn-Stokes, A. and Routh, D. (1994) 'Intergroup contact between professional groups: two evaluation studies', *Journal of Community and Applied Social Psychology*, vol 4, pp 347-63.

Hind, M., Norman, I.J., Cooper, S., Gill, E., Hilton, R., Judd, P. and Jones, S.C. (2003) 'Interprofessional perceptions of health care students', *Journal of Interprofessional Care*, vol 17, pp 21-34.

HM Government (2010) *Working together to safeguard children: A guide to inter-agency working to safeguard and promote the welfare of children*, London: HM Government.

Horbar, J., Rogowski, J. and Plsek, P. (2001) 'Collaborative quality improvement for neonatal intensive care', *Pediatrics*, vol 107, pp 14-22.

House of Commons Health Committee (2009) *Patient safety: Sixth report of session 2008-09*, London: The Stationery Office.

Hudson, B. (2000) 'Inter-agency collaboration: a sceptical view', in A. Brechin, H. Brown, and M.A. Eby (eds) *Critical practice in health and social care*, Milton Keynes: Open University Press.

Humphris, D. and Hean, S. (2004) 'Educating the future workforce: building the evidence about interprofessional learning', *Journal of Health Services Research and Policy*, vol 9, pp 24-7.

Hylin, U., Nyholm, H., Mattiasson, A.-C. and Ponzer, S. (2007) 'Interprofessional training in clinical practice on a training ward for healthcare students: a two-year follow-up', *Journal of Interprofessional Care*, vol 21, pp 277-88.

Interprofessional Education Collaborative Expert Panel (2011) *Core competencies for interprofessional collaborative practice: Report of an expert panel*, Washington, DC: Interprofessional Collaborative

IOM (Institute of Medicine) (2015) *Measuring the impact of interprofessional education on collaborative practice and patient outcomes*, Washington, DC: The National Academies Press (http://iom. nationalacademies.org/Reports/2015/Impact-of-IPE.aspx).

Jelphs, K., Dickinson, H. and Miller, R. (2016) *Working in teams* (2nd edn), Better Partnership Working series, Bristol: Policy Press.

Jupp, B. (2000) *Working together: Creating a better environment for cross-sector partnerships*, London: Demos.

Ker, J., Mole, L. and Bradley, P. (2003) 'Early introduction of interprofessional learning: a simulated ward environment', *Medical Teacher*, vol 37, pp 248-55.

Kirkpatrick, D.I. (1967) 'Evaluation of training', in R. Craig and I. Bittel (eds) *Training and development handbook*, New York, NY: McGraw-Hill.

Knapp, M., Bennett, N., Plumb, J. and Robinson, J. (2000) 'Community-based quality improvement education for health professions: balancing benefits for communities and students', *Journal of Interprofessional Care*, vol 14, pp 119-30.

Knowles, M.S. (1990) *The adult learner: A neglected species*, Houston, TX: Gulf Publishing.

Kohn, L.T., Corrigan, J.M. and Donaldson M.S. (eds) (1999) *To err is human: Building a safer health system*, Committee on Quality of Health Care in America, Washington, DC: Institute of Medicine.

Kotter, J.P. (1995) 'Leading change: why transformation efforts fail', *Harvard Business Review*, pp 59-67.

Kreindler, S., Dowd, D., Starr, N.D. and Gottschalk, T. (2012) 'Silos and social identity: the social identity approach as a framework for understanding and overcoming divisions in health care', *The Milbank Quarterly*, vol 90, pp 347-74.

Kuehn, A.F. (1998) 'Collaborative health professional education: An interdisciplinary mandate for the third millennium', in T.J. Sullivan (ed) *Collaboration: A health care imperative*, New York: McGraw-Hill, pp 419-65.

Kwan, D., Barker, K., Zubin, A., Chatalalsingh, C., Grdisa, V., Langlois, S. et al (2006) 'Effectiveness of a faculty development program on interprofessional education: a randomized controlled trial', *Journal of Interprofessional Care*, vol 20, pp 314-16.

Ladden, M.D., Bednash, G., Stevens, D.P. and Moore, G.T. (2006) 'Educating interprofessional learners for quality, safety and systems improvement', *Journal of Interprofessional Care*, vol 20, pp 497-505.

Laming, H. (2003) *The Victoria Climbié Inquiry: Report of an inquiry*, London: The Stationery Office.

Laming, W. (2009) *The protection of children in England: A progress report*, London: The Stationery Office.

Lawlis, T.R., Anson, J. and Greenfield, D. (2014) 'Barriers and enablers that influence sustainable interprofessional education: a literature review', *Journal of Interprofessional Care*, vol 28, no 4, pp 305-10.

Leff, J., Sharpley, M., Chisholm, D., Bell, R. and Gamble, C. (2001) 'Training CPNs in schizophrenia family work: a study of clinical and economic outcomes for patients and relatives', *Journal of Mental Health*, vol 10, pp 189-97.

Leutz, W. (1999) 'Five laws for integrating medical and social services: lessons from the United States and the United Kingdom', *The Milbank Quarterly*, vol 77, no 1, pp 77-110.

Levin, E. (2004) *Involving service users and carers in social work education*, London: Social Care Institute for Excellence.

Lidskog, M., Löfmark, A. and Ahlström, G. (2007) 'Interprofessional education on a training ward for older people: students' conceptions of nurses, occupational therapists and social workers', *Journal of Interprofessional Care*, vol 21, pp 387-99.

Lindqvist, S., Duncan, A., Shepstone, L., Watts, F. and Pearce, S. (2005) 'Case-based learning in cross-professional groups – the development of a pre-registration interprofessional learning programme', *Journal of Interprofessional Care*, vol 19, pp 509-20.

Luecht, R.M., Madsen, M.K., Taugher, M.P. and Petterson, B.J. (1990) 'Assessing professional perceptions: design and validation of an interdisciplinary education perception scale', *Journal of Allied Health*, spring, pp 181-91.

McCallin, A. (2001) 'Interdisciplinary practice – a matter of teamwork: an integrated literature review', *Journal of Clinical Nursing*, vol 10, pp 419-28.

McFadyen, A.K., Maclaren, M. and Webster, V. (2007) 'The Interdisciplinary Education Perception Scale (IEPS): An alternative remodelled subscale structure and its reliability', *Journal of Interprofessional Care*, vol 21, pp 433-43.

McFadyen, A.K., Webster, V. and Maclaren, W.M. (2006) 'The test-retest reliability of a revised version of the Readiness for Interprofessional Learning Scale (RIPLS)', *Journal of Interprofessional Care*, vol 20, pp 633-9.

McFadyen, A.K., Webster, V., Maclaren, W. and O'Neill, M. (2010) 'Interprofessional attitudes and perceptions: Results from a longitudinal controlled trial of preregistration health and social care students in Scotland', *Journal of Interprofessional Care*, vol 24, pp 549-64.

Mandy, A., Milton, C. and Mandy, P. (2004) 'Professional stereotyping and interprofessional education', *Learning in Health and Social Care*, vol 3, pp 154-70.

Makino, T., Shinozaki, H., Hayashi, K., Lee, B., Matsui, H., Kururi, N. et al (2012) 'Attitudes toward interprofessional healthcare teams: A comparison between undergraduate students and alumni', *Journal of Interprofessional Care*, vol 26, no 2, pp 100-7.

Meads, G. (2007) *Walk the talk: Sustainable change in post 2000 interprofessional learning and development*, London: Department of Health.

Miller, C., Ross, N. and Freeman, M. (1999) *Shared learning and clinical teamwork: New directions in education for multiprofessional practice*, London: ENB.

Mohaupt, J., van Soeren, M., Andrusyszyn, M-A., MacMillan K., Devlin-Cop, S. and Reeves, S. (2012) 'Understanding interprofessional relationships by the use of contact theory', *Journal of Interprofessional Care*, vol 26, pp 370-5.

Morey, J., Simon, R. and Jay, G. (2002) 'Error reduction and performance improvement in the emergency department through formal teamwork training: evaluation results of the MedTeams Project', *Health Services Research*, vol 37, pp 1553-81.

Morgan, A. and Jones, D. (2009) 'Perceptions of service user and carer involvement in healthcare education and impact on students' knowledge and practice: A literature review', *Medical Teacher*, vol 31, pp 82-95.

Morrison, S., Boohan, M., Jenkins, J. and Moutray, M. (2003) 'Facilitating undergraduate interprofessional education in health care: comparing classroom and clinical learning for nursing and medical students', *Learning in Health and Social Care*, vol 2, pp 92-104.

Nasmith, L. and Oandasan, I. (2003) *Interdisciplinary education in primary health care: Moving beyond tokenism*, Calgary, Alberta: College of Family Physicians of Canada Family Medicine Forum.

Nickol, D.R. (2015) 'Interprofessional education: what's now, and what's next?', *Journal of Interprofessional Education & Practice*, vol 1, pp 1-2.

O'Halloran, C., Hean, S., Humphris, D. and Macleod-Clark, J. (2006) 'Developing common learning: the New Generation Project undergraduate curriculum model', *Journal of Interprofessional Care*, vol 20, pp 12-28.

Oandasan, I. and Reeves, S. (2005) 'Key elements of interprofessional education. Part 2: Factors, processes and outcomes', *Journal of Interprofessional Care*, vol 19, pp 39-48.

Oliver, D., Wittenberg-Lyles, E.M. and Day, M. (2007) 'Measuring interdisciplinary perceptions of collaboration on hospice teams', *American Journal of Hospice and Palliative Medicine*, vol 24, no 1, pp 49-53.

Parsell, G. and Bligh, J. (1999) 'The development of a questionnaire to assess the readiness of healthcare students for interprofessional learning', *Medical Education*, vol 33, pp 95-100.

Parsell, G., Spalding, R. and Bligh, J. (1998) 'Shared goals, shared learning: evaluation of a multiprofessional course for undergraduate students', *Medical Education*, vol 32, pp 304-11.

Patsios, D. and Carpenter, J. (2010) 'Organisation of interagency training for safeguarding children in England: a case study using realistic evaluation', *International Journal of Integrated Care*, vol 10, 16 November, pp 1-12.

Pawson, R. and Tilley, N. (1997) *Realistic evaluation*, London: Sage Publications.

Payne, M. (2000) *Teamwork in multiprofessional care*, Basingstoke: Macmillan.

Peck, E. and Dickinson, H. (2010) 'Pursuing legitimacy: conceptualising and developing leaders' performances', *Leadership & Organization Development Journal*, vol 31, no 7, pp 630-42.

Pettigrew, T.F. (1998) 'Intergroup contact theory', *Annual Review of Psychology*, vol 49, pp 65-85.

Pollard, K., Miers, M. and Gilchrist, M. (2004) 'Collaborative learning for collaborative working? Initial findings from a longitudinal study of health and social care students', *Health and Social Care in the Community*, vol 12, pp 346-58.

Pollard, K., Miers, M. and Gilchrist, M. (2005) 'Second year scepticism: pre-qualifying health and social care students' midpoint self-assessment, attitudes and perceptions concerning interprofessional learning and working', *Journal of Interprofessional Care*, vol 19, pp 251-68.

Pollard, K., Fletcher, I., Martin, M. and Hughes, M. (2014) 'The University of the West of England', in H. Barr, M. Helme and L. D'Avray, *Developing interprofessional education in health and social care courses in the United Kingdom*, London: Higher Education Academy, pp 75-83.

Pollard, K., Miers, M., Gilchrist, M. and Sayers, A. (2006) 'A comparison of interprofessional perceptions and working relationships among health and social care students: the results of a 3-year intervention', *Health and Social Care in the Community*, vol 14, pp 541-52.

Ponzer, S., Hylin, U., Kusoffsky, A., Lauffs, M., Lonka, K., Mattiasson, A. and Nordstrom, G. (2004) 'Interprofessional training in the context of clinical practice: goals and students' perceptions on clinical education wards', *Medical Education*, vol 38, pp 727-36.

Rees, D. and Johnson, R. (2007) 'All together now? Staff views and experiences of a pre-qualifying interprofessional curriculum', *Journal of Interprofessional Care*, vol 21, pp 543-55.

Reeves, S. (2000) 'Community-based interprofessional education for medical, nursing and dental students', *Health and Social Care in the Community*, vol 8, pp 269-76.

Reeves, S. (2001) 'A systematic review of the effects of interprofessional education on staff involved in the care of adults with mental health problems', *Journal of Psychiatric and Mental Health Nursing*, vol 8, pp 533-42.

Reeves, S. and Hean, S. (2013) 'Why we need theory to help us better understand the nature of interprofessional education, practice and care', *Journal of Interprofessional Care*, vol 27, pp 1-3.

Reeves, S. and Freeth, D. (2002) 'The London training ward: an innovative interprofessional learning initiative', *Journal of Interprofessional Care*, vol 16, pp 41-52.

Reeves, S. and Freeth, D. (2006) 'Re-examining the evaluation of interprofessional education for community mental health teams with a different lens: understanding presage, process and product factors', *Journal of Psychiatric and Mental Health Nursing*, vol 13, pp 765-70.

Reeves, S. and Hean, S. (2013) 'Why we need theory to help us better understand the nature of interprofessional education, practice and care', *Journal of Interprofessional Care*, vol 27, pp 1-3.

Reeves, S. and Sully, P. (2007) 'Interprofessional education for practitioners working with the survivors of violence: exploring early and longer-term outcomes on practice', *Journal of Interprofessional Care*, vol 21, pp 401-12.

Reeves, S., Freeth, D., McCrorie, P. and Perry, D. (2002) 'Teamworking "it teaches you what to expect in the future...": interprofessional learning on a training ward for medical, nursing, occupational therapy and physiotherapy students', *Medical Education*, vol 36, pp 337-44.

Reeves, S., Perrier, L., Goldman, J., Freeth, D. and Zwarenstein, M. (2013) 'Interprofessional education: effects on professional practice and healthcare outcomes (update)', *Cochrane Database System Review*, 3: CD002213.

Robson, C. (1993) *Real world research: Resources for real world scientists and practitioner-researchers*, Oxford: Blackwell Publishers.

Rogowski, J., Horbar, J., Plsek, P., Schurmann Baker, L., Deterding, J., Edwards, W.H. et al (2001) 'Economic implications of neonatal intensive care unit collaborative quality improvement', *Pediatrics*, vol 107, p 29.

Romanow Commission (2002) *Commission on the future of health care in Canada*, Ottawa: Health Canada (www.hc-sc.gc.ca/hcs-sss/com/fed/romanow/index-eng.php).

Rothbart, M. and John, O.P. (1985) 'Social cognition and behavioural episodes: A cognitive analysis of the effects of intergroup contact', *Journal of Social Issues*, vol 41, pp 81-104.

Rummery, K. and Glendinning, C. (2000) *Primary care and social services: Developing new partnerships for older people*, Abingdon: Radcliffe Medical Press.

Rushmer, R. (2005) 'Blurred boundaries damage inter-professional working', *Nurse Researcher*, vol 12, pp 74-85.

Rushmer, R. and Pallis, G. (2002) 'Inter-professional working: the wisdom of integrated working and the disaster of blurred boundaries', *Public Money and Management*, pp 59-66.

Schön, D.A. (1987) *Educating the reflective practitioners: Towards a new design for teaching and learning in the profession*, San Francisco, CA: Jossey-Bass.

Scott, J. (2003) *A fair day's pay: A guide to benefits, service user involvement and payments*, London: Mental Health Foundation.

Secretary of State for Health (2001) *The report of the Public Inquiry into Children's Heart Surgery at the Bristol Royal Infirmary 1984-1995: Learning from Bristol*, London: The Stationery Office.

Spry, E. (2006) 'All together for health', *Student BMJ*, vol 14, p 2.

Steketee, S., Forman, D., Dunston, R. et al (2014) 'Interprofessional health education in Australia: Three research projects informing curriculum renewal and development', *Applied Nursing Research*, vol 27, no 2, pp 115-20.

Steven, A., Dickinson, C. and Pearson, P. (2007) 'Practice-based interprofessional education: looking into the black box', *Journal of Interprofessional Care*, vol 21, pp 251-64.

Strasser, D.C., Falconer. J.A., Stevens, A.B. et al (2008) 'Team training and stroke rehabilitation outcomes: a cluster randomized trial', *Archives of Physical Medicine & Rehabilitation*, vol 89, no 1, pp 10-15.

Stumpf, S.H. and Clark, J.Z. (1999) 'The promise and pragmatism of inter-disciplinary education', *Journal of Allied Health*, vol 28, pp 30-2.

Sullivan, H. and Skelcher, C. (2002) *Working across boundaries: Collaboration in public services*, Basingstoke: Palgrave.

Szasz, G. (1969) 'Interprofessional education in the health sciences', *Milbank Memorial Fund Quarterly*, vol 47, pp 449-75.

Tajfel, H. and Turner, J.C. (1986) 'The social identity theory of intergroup behaviour', in S. Worschel and W. Austin (eds) *Psychology of intergroup relations*, Chicago, IL: Nelson-Hall.

Takahashi, H.E. and Kinoshita, M. (2015) 'Formation of the Japan Association for Interprofessional Education', in D. Forman, M. Jones and J. Thistlethwaite (eds) *Leadership and collaboration: Further developments for interprofessional education*, Basingstoke: Palgrave Macmillan, pp 47-70.

Tew, J., Gell, C. and Foster, S. (2004) *Learning from experience: Involving service users and carers in mental health education and training*, Nottingham: Higher Education Academy/National Institute for Mental Health in England/NHA Workforce Development Confederation.

Thannhauser, J., Russell-Mayhew, S. and Scott, C. (2010) 'Measures of interprofessional education and collaboration', *Journal of Interprofessional Care*, vol 24, pp 336-49.

Thistlethwaite, J. (2012) 'Interprofessional education: A review of context, learning and the research agenda', *Medical Education*, vol 46, pp 58-70.

Thomas, J., Clarke, B., Pollard, K. and Miers, M. (2007) 'Facilitating interprofessional enquiry-based learning: dilemmas and strategies', *Journal of Interprofessional Care*, vol 21, pp 463-5.

Towle, A. (2007) 'Involving patients in the education of health care professionals', *Journal of Health Services Research and Policy*, vol 12, pp 1-2.

Treadwell, M., Franck, L. and Vichinsky, E. (2002) 'Using quality improvement strategies to predict pain assessment', *International Journal for Quality in Health Care*, vol 14, pp 39-47.

Tucker, K., Wakefield, A., Boggis, C., Lawson, M., Roberts, T. and Gooch, J. (2003) 'Learning together: clinical skills teaching for medical and nursing students', *Medical Education*, vol 37, pp 630-7.

Tunstall-Pedoe, S., Rink, E. and Hilton, S. (2003) 'Student attitudes to undergraduate interprofessional education', *Journal of Interprofessional Care*, vol 17, pp 161-72.

Turner, P., Sheldon, F., Coles, C., Mountford, B., Hillier, R., Radway, P. and Wee, B. (2000) 'Listening to and learning from the family carer's story: an innovative approach in interprofessional education', *Journal of Interprofessional Care*, vol 14, pp 387-95.

Wakefield, A., Cooke, S. and Boggis, C. (2003) 'Learning together: use of simulated patients with nursing and medical students for breaking bad news', *International Journal of Palliative Nursing*, vol 9, pp 32-8.

Watanabe, H. and Koizumi, M. (2010) *Advanced initiatives in interprofessional education in Japan*, Tokyo: Springer.

WHO (World Health Organization) (1988) *Learning together to work together for health. Report of a WHO study group on multiprofessional education for health personnel: The team approach*, Technical Report Series 769, Geneva: WHO.

WHO (2010) *Framework for action on interprofessional education and collaborative practice*, Health Professions Networks/Nursing & Midwifery/Human Resources for Health (WHO/HRH/HPN/10.3), Geneva: WHO (http://apps.who.int/iris/bitstream/10665/70185/1/WHO_HRH_HPN_10.3_eng.pdf).

Wistow, G. and Waddington, E. (2006) 'Learning from doing: implications of the Barking and Dagenham experiences for integrating health and social care', *Journal of Integrated Care*, vol 14, pp 8-18.

Wykurz, G. and Kelly, D. (2002) 'Developing the role of patients as teachers: literature review', *British Medical Journal*, vol 325, pp 818-21.

Zwarenstein, M., Reeves, S. and Perrier, L. (2005) 'Effectiveness of pre-licensure interprofessional education and post-licensure collaborative interventions', *Journal of Interprofessional Care*, vol 3, pp 148-65.

Zwarenstein, M., Goldman, J. and Reeves, S. (2009) 'Interprofessional collaboration: Effects of practice-based interventions on professional practice and healthcare outcomes', *Cochrane Database of Systematic Reviews*, 3:CD000072. doi:10.1002/14651858.CD000072. pub2.

Zwarenstein, M., Reeves, S., Barr, H., Hammick, M., Koppel, I. and Atkins, J. (2000) *Interprofessional education: Effects on professional practice and health care outcomes*, Cochrane Database of Systematic Reviews.

Index